Intermittent Fasting For Women and Ketogenic-Diet & Intermittent-Fasting

2 Manuscripts

The Ideal Weight Loss Guide for Men and Women Who Are Keto Beginners, Including Rapid Fat Loss and Increased Health.

By: Amy Moore

Intermittent-Fasting and

Ketogenic-Diet

An Easy, Beginner Weight Loss Challenge for Men and Women to Maximize Healthy Weight Loss With Keto

By: Amy Moore

Table Of Contents

Introduction

   WHY FOLLOW THIS DIET

   CHAPTER ONE: WHAT DOES INTERMITTENT FASTING MEAN?

   HISTORICAL DEVELOPMENT OF INTERMITTENT FASTING
   TESTIMONIES REGARDING INTERMITTENT FASTING

   CHAPTER TWO: WHY INTERMITTENT FASTING WORKS

   MYTHS/ MISCONCEPTIONS REGARDING INTERMITTENT FASTING

   CHAPTER THREE: WHAT DO WE MEAN BY KETOGENIC DIET?

   THE HISTORICAL DEVELOPMENT OF KETOGENIC DIET
   TESTIMONIES ACKNOWLEDGING THE EFFICACY OF THE KETOGENIC DIET
   How I eat

   CHAPTER FOUR: WHY THE KETOGENIC DIET WORKS

   MISCONCEPTIONS AND WRONG THOUGHTS ABOUT KETOGENIC DIET

YOU CAN CONSUME AS MUCH FAT AS YOU WANT
KETOSIS AND KETOACIDOSIS ARE TOTALLY THE SAME
KETOGENIC DIET IS A HIGH PROTEIN DIET
FASTING IS A REQUIREMENT FOR KETO DIET
KETO DIET IS ALCOHOL RESISTANCE
KETOGENIC DIET IS ONLY GOOD FOR WEIGHT LOSS
THE BRAIN NEEDS SUGAR TO FUNCTION

CHAPTER FIVE: WHY YOU SHOULD ENGAGE IN KETOGENIC DIET AND INTERMITTENT FASTING FOR WEIGHT LOSS

OTHER WEIGHT LOSS PROGRAMS THAT YOU CAN REPLACE WITH THE KETOGENIC DIET AND INTERMITTENT FASTING

Going to the gym

Use of herbal medicines and drugs

Jogging and other forms of exercise

Employing the use of work-out videos

CHAPTER SIX: BENEFITS OF INTERMITTENT FASTING

1. IMPROVES FAT BURNING
2. IT INCREASES WEIGHT AND BODY FAT LOSS
3. IT INCREASES YOUR ENERGY LEVEL
4. IT LOWERS SUGAR LEVELS AND BLOOD INSULIN

5. IT IMPROVES MENTAL CLARITY AND CONCENTRATION
6. IT REVERSES TYPE TWO DIABETES
BENEFITS OF THE KETOGENIC DIET

CHAPTER SEVEN: DIFFERENT TYPES AND KINDS OF INTERMITTENT FASTING

DIFFERENT TYPES OF THE KETOGENIC DIET

CHAPTER EIGHT: CHOOSING THE PERFECT INTERMITTENT FASTING FOR YOU

CHOOSING THE PERFECT KETOGENIC DIET
THE STANDARD KETOGENIC DIET
THE TARGETED KETOGENIC DIET
THE CYCLIC KETOGENIC DIET
THE HIGH PROTEIN KETOGENIC DIET
THE PROTEIN SPARING MODIFIED FAST

CHAPTER NINE: WHAT TO EAT AND NOT TO EAT

WATCH THE FATS YOU EAT
DRINK A LOT OF WATER
ALCOHOL INTAKE
JUNK AND LATE NIGHT SNACK
THINGS TO DO AND THINGS NOT TO DO
DO EXERCISE WHEN OPPORTUNE
DO WATCH YOUR CALORIES
DO AVOID FAST FOOD

CHAPTER TEN: TIPS ON KETOGENIC DIET

CLEAR CARBOHYDRATES FROM YOUR KITCHEN
HAVE KETOGENIC SNACKS AT HAND
BUY A FOOD SCALE
EXERCISE FREQUENTLY
TRY INTERMITTENT FASTING
INCLUDE COCONUT OIL INTO YOUR DIET
FREQUENTLY ASKED QUESTIONS AND ANSWERS TO THEM
Can pregnant women do the ketogenic diet?
At what level should my ketones be during ketosis?
Can I develop muscles while doing my ketogenic diet?
How long can I be on the ketogenic diet?
How long does it take to be in ketosis?

CONCLUSION

Introduction

Why Follow This Diet

Unlike what a lot of people say about how easy it is to lose weight and stay healthy and fit, losing weight can be very difficult and hard even when one is trying so hard.

It can be especially frustrating trying to fit into the clothes one got a few years back. Even if an output costs so much, it can all go to waste if it does not fit one after a short period of time.

People have various views regarding weight loss, staying healthy and fit but it is quite difficult most of the time.

The challenge of getting fit and healthy, losing weight is quite excruciating.

One may have gone through several weight loss therapies, challenges, and so on but all seem to no avail. The reason most of the weight loss therapies are hard to stick to is because of our schedule, the type of job you have, responsibilities you carry and many other factors.

These therapies and diets have also crashed most of your energy. For example, I can't imagine myself working in a factory and I have to be on a strict diet which crashes my energy and reduces my work efficiency.

Another important reason that studies have shown that makes weight loss quite difficult is due to other failed therapies an individual has gone through. You might have engaged in some diets that failed, that is, there was no result. This is quite discouraging.

Now, what if I tell you that there is a way that weight loss can be made efficient, easy, and it would bring out active and positive results? It might be hard to believe due to previous experiences but research has shown that through intermittent fasting and the ketogenic diet, weight loss, staying healthy and fit has been made more efficient.

Research and studies have revealed that intermittent fasting has a great effect on weight and body fat loss. It also lowers the blood insulin and sugar levels. Intermittent fasting also lowers blood cholesterol, and it reduces inflammation. It has also been revealed that it activates cellular cleansing by stimulating autophagy [this discovery was awarded the 2016 Nobel Prize in medicine]. Activation of intermittent fasting prevents Alzheimer's disease and it also elongates the lifespan of an individual.

Ketogenic diet on the other hand has been proven to be better than most diets at helping people with obesity, high blood pressure, high blood sugar level, heart disease, fatty liver disease, cancer, migraines, Alzheimer's disease, Parkinson's disease, Type 2 diabetes, Type 1 diabetes, and so on. Even though you are not really at risk from any of the conditions listed above, the ketogenic diet has been said to be very helpful for you. Some of the few benefits that a vast number of people experience include better brain function, improved and good body composition, a high increase in energy, a rapid decrease in inflammation.

As you can observe, the ketogenic diet has a vast and enormous catalog of benefits, but the question is, is it any better than other diets?

Many people have had various testimonies, all attesting to the effectiveness of intermittent fasting and ketogenic fasting.

Below is a wonderful success story of a woman who dropped 50 pounds in 4 months: 'I did not feel anywhere near as bloated or sick. I felt healthier on the inside because I was not putting bad foods in my body... It has also seriously improved my anxiety and depression because I do not feel the way I used to feel before, I feel elated and wonderful.'

Having backed up the efficacy of intermittent fasting and the ketogenic diet, it should be pointed out that a doctor's prescription should be taken into attention.

Many questions come to mind like, 'what makes the ketogenic diet distinct from other diets? 'Why should it be taken seriously? 'Is the intermittent fast not another word for starvation?'

Those questions would be answered in this book.

Chapter One: What Does Intermittent Fasting Mean?

The word fasting literarily means to abstain from all foods. To a layman, it could mean starvation, which is not really the exact meaning. Fasting is the process of intentional abstinence from food. It can also be the abstinence from certain types of foods due to religious beliefs.

To be fasting derives from a motive, that is, you are chasing after something. You can do it due to some certain religious beliefs. It can also be done to achieve weight loss and to stay healthy and fit. This might sound like an irony to most people. How can fasting which implies starvation keep my body fit and healthy? Well, research has shown that the act of fasting can be an advantage to the human system.

The word intermittent means occurring at time intervals. It can also mean something or activity not happening continuously or steadily.

Now, 'intermittent fasting' is the act of abstaining from food on an irregular schedule.

Intermittent fasting is a major tool for weight reduction and healthy living. Intermittent fasting is currently one of the current most popular health and fitness programs which keep one fit and healthy.

Intermittent fasting can be defined as an eating pattern that cycle between periods of fasting and eating. In this accord, it cannot be referred or said to be a diet, it is more like an eating pattern. The most common intermittent fasting routines involve daily 16-hour fasting or 24 hours fasts, twice per week.

Historical Development Of Intermittent Fasting

Fasting has been in existence for ages, it is a practice that has been carried out throughout human evolution. Ancient hunter-gatherers did not have malls, supermarkets, refrigerators, freezers for food preservation. They did not have foods that lasted year round. Sometimes they could not find anything to eat. As a result, man evolved to be able to function without foods for an extended period of time.

It can be said that there was no time in man's history that fasting was not practiced. In every written antiquity about cultures, geography, and religions, there is a cogent and important mention of fasting.

In ancient India, ancient Greece and ancient Egypt, fasting was used as a very useful tool in the curative strengthening of the spiritual cycle and spirit of man, and preventive health concerns.

In the Greek culture, contemporary fasting is totally different from the way the predecessors practiced it. In this present day, animal products are to be abstained from, while during the time of the predecessors, all foods were to be abstained from and only water was taken. It is recorded that one of the fathers of mathematics and a great philosopher Pythagoras [580-500 B.C.], systematically starved for 40 days with the conception or belief that it rapidly increases the mental perception, innovativeness, and creativity- a notion that the scientists of today have proven to be exactly and accurately true. It is also well-recorded that Pythagoras and his diligent followers were strict and adhering vegetarians.

Plato [427-347 B.C], who was a devoted follower and disciple of Socrates, had divided medicine into true and false, the true being that which gives health, which included fasting.

Hippocrates [460-357BC], the renowned father of modern medicine, was the one who invented and created the Mediterranean diet and also removed fasting from the realm of philosophy into a medical necessity. He made mention of the following concerning fasting for a sick person. Below is only a little extract: 'The addition of food should be rarer, since it is often useful to completely take it away while the patient can withstand it, until the force of the disease reaches its maturity. If the body is cleared, the more you feed it the more it will be harmed. When a patient is fed too richly, the disease is fed as well... excess is against nature.'

The primitive Greeks had made an observation that the periods by which they fast would cause the seizures of an epileptic to become less occurring and less severe. Anticonvulsant drugs were not in existence until the 1950s. The Greeks also believed that fasting improves a person's cognitive alertness.

Fasting was also mentioned in the Bible and it had discussed the events of several 40 days concurrent fasting including those of Elijah and of Jesus.

Fasting was also in view in Islamic history; Muslims also fast from sunrise to sunset during the holy period of Ramadan. It is the best studied of the fasting periods. It is quite different from any other fasting periods in that fluids are also forbidden. They also undergo a period of mild dehydration, since eating is allowed before the sun rises and after the sun sets.

Fasting was practiced through the history of man; it evolved alongside man. Around the 14th century, fasting was duly practiced by St Catherine of Siena.

If we take a very critical look, fasting has become rapidly and increasingly practiced over the last few decades, but the question is, why the sudden change? It is what I would like to call the enlightenment; people are beginning to see that there is more to fasting than being devoted; the act of fasting has health and medical benefits.

Testimonies Regarding Intermittent Fasting

Testimonies regarding Intermittent fasting also known as IF are in various forms because people who practiced it actually saw results which were quite a surprise on their path.

We, humans, have been in the habit of practicing intermittent fasting since the dawn of time, but it has now yielded to be an incredible and very useful tool in the fitness world.

The beauty in intermittent fasting is that an individual can eat whatever he/she dims fit because it is certainly not a diet; it is an eating pattern

You can definitely be a ketogenic diet if you deem fit but it is really advisable in order to get greater results.

Some people find themselves consuming the same amount of calories with intermittent fasting or without intermittent fasting, a vast number of people observe a decrease in calorie intake, the reason being that it is easier to get full faster in a shorter period of time. Intermittent fasting is true to all, neither does it lie because some women have testified to the efficacy of its effectiveness and how it has incredibly transformed and refurbished their lives. Below are testimonies of various people on how intermittent has transformed their lives and have given them a reason to smile again:

These testimonies are taken from various websites and will be referenced as footnotes, and also at the end of the book.

A 23-year-old lady, Rachel said, "*I do a lot of comparisons photos, it keeps me motivated. It is crazy to think I have lost 63+ pounds in a number of weeks and still have 5 more months to go until my goal of one year!*"

Another lady Sharon said, "*14 weeks of intermittent fasting... 18 lbs gone.*"

Lynn said, "*I could not even smile right because I was so focused on holding it in.*"

Suma said, "*Down 56 lbs! It has been exactly one year since I started and it has been beyond life changing for me.*

In one year since adopting an intermittent fasting lifestyle, I have:

- Weight loss of 56.4 lbs
- Went down 12% body fat
- Dropped 50.5 inches around my body
- Gone from a size 14 to 4.
- Moved from being categorized as 'obese' to 'normal weight'

according to my BMI
- No more issues with sleep apnea, being pre-diabetic or high blood pressure.

So what is next for me? Now that I have hit my first big goal of losing 55 lbs, I'm excited to layer in weightlifting with intermittent fasting. My goal is to stop looking at the scale and instead focus on increasing lean muscle mass and reduce body fat."[1]

Martha said, "I loved the dress I was wearing. I thought I looked great and I actually wore it to events I was invited to. I bought the dress because I thought it was flattering for my shape and I thought it had my tummy…until I saw a picture of myself that was taken.

I was pushing 76-77 kg in the picture I saw. I was big, unhealthy and very unhappy. I hid my real feelings behind that fake smile and I was an emotional eater. I was lazy and at this stage had stopped going to the gym, my diet was high in carbs and sugar. I was drinking up to 4 cans of Pepsi in a day and eating takeout a couple of times in a week. I really didn't have any plans to change my lifestyle.

What was my wakeup call? A letter from the NDSS [National Diabetes Service Scheme] reminding me that I needed to sit a diabetes test. It was my second reminder. I ignored the first one, but for some reason, reading the second reminder scared the crap out of me, I lost my father to advanced renal failure and I refused to go that road. I needed to sort my shit out and get healthy and lose weight. So I did. I have lost 8 kilos since November when I started a ketogenic lifestyle and I am motivated to lose more. I am the key to my own success. If I don't remain positive and motivated, I will go back to my old ways and I absolutely refuse to be that girl again. Do not just read my success story, become the author of your own."[2]

Stella said, "Thank God for macro counting, intermittent fasting, still a very long way to go."

Jpanzini said, "Have a long way to go still, but proud of where I came from...all thanks to intermittent fasting."

Stacy said, "Back in May I started a challenge with 15 other friends, I was 158 lbs.

The first month I lost about 3 lbs and since I was drinking and eating my face off each weekend, I was happy with that. At least the weight was going down. I was working out about 4-5 times a week. The process was so slow! Mid-August I had spent an exhausting week reading/watching/listening to everything I could learn about intermittent fasting and jumped in. I am now in my 9th week and weigh about 142. I have lost 12 lbs so far, about 1lb in a week, but I am very happy with that! This is what has happened in the last 9 weeks:

I lost 4lbs right away but still losing an average of 1lb per week

I workout less. 3 times a week, maybe 4. Depends. I no longer beat myself up if I don't.

I am what they call the mix between 20/4 and "eat stop eat" I do 2-24 hour fast a week and on other days I have a 4-hour window. Saturday I enjoy breakfast and eat whatever during football till 6 pm then stops eating to get a jump on the week.

I have a ton of energy and I am getting things done. So much extra time when I am not planning out meals and have food all day long. This exists- you probably don't even know how much food weighs us down during the day

I know that while fasting behind my body is repairing itself from inside. It is not using all its energy digesting so now my body focuses on repair. So on the days I am discouraged I just keep going!

This is a lifestyle now for me. I am in it for good!

Intermittent fasting saved me."[3]

Amber said, "I began slowly gaining weight around 10 years ago. I attribute this to a time of extreme stress which caused me to quit caring for myself physically. Prior to this, I had always been what most would consider thin. It took a few years for the weight gain to become visible to others, and even then, most would not have considered it extreme. It wasn't until about 2015 that it really became noticeable.

I rationalized my weight gain, however, and consoled myself with the comparison to others. On occasion, I would encounter a picture that I was not able to throw out, and I would be confronted with the truth. I had gone from wearing sizes 4-6 to wearing 12-14's at the height of my weight gain. I had no idea how much I weighed, as my scale had broken years before and I had never replaced it.

In the summer of 2017 I made a trip to Bed Bath and Beyond and on a whim, I decided to step on one of their operating scales. Before I did, I guessed that at 5' 7.5" that my weight would be in the 160-pound range. I knew that wasn't great, but in my mind, I could justify it. So, I stepped on the scale and it said 188.8 pounds. I stood in the store in front of two other women and wept.

In a moment of clarity, I decided to get it together and buy the scale. I went home and had a total pity party. "How could this happen? When did this happen?" I knew the answer to both questions. I had done all of it.

The next day I got up and resolved to fix the problem that I had created. I was the only one capable of digging myself out of the hole. I began by just watching what I ate, walking every day, and focusing on healthy fats and portion control. It wasn't long after that I began a HI-IT workout three times a week. I lost weight with this approach, but an odd thing happened... I found that when I got up in the morning that I no longer wanted to eat breakfast. In fact, I resented being told that I must.

At some point on my Facebook feed, I started getting information about Intermittent Fasting from various sources. One that I remember suggesting that women should fast 12-14 hours, then have their first meal. I dabbled with that for some time and felt great doing it.

It wasn't until November of 2017 that Delay, Don't Deny: Intermittent Fasting Support showed up on my Facebook feed. I was intrigued and joined the group. Within a day or two, I had purchased the book and read it in an evening. I've never looked back since.

Starting in November I began fasting 16 hours a day. I quickly within a couple of weeks went to 19:5 and then shortly thereafter went to One Meal a Day or OMAD. It felt so natural and freeing. In the middle of December of 2017, my husband joined me in OMAD and we are still OMAD to date.

My husband has lost 30. In addition to the weight loss, both of us have a renewed lease on life and an appreciation for each other. I no longer have to pick my clothes based on what I need to cover up, but rather what I should showcase. At 48, that is a definite WIN. :) My husband has found increased endurance for his physically demanding job as a builder at 57.

Neither one of us plans on ever going back to eating as we did before.

Intermittent Fasting is now our lifestyle."[4]

Darras said, "Imagine you have to attend a party or you are invited on a family dinner and you cannot eat because you don't want to push yourself 2 weeks back by eating all those foods that you have been avoiding for months. The worst part, it is even harder to deal with people and make them realize that you are on a diet. Intermittent fasting has saved my life, I once felt dejected and sad about how I have become but thanks to intermittent fasting I feel and very optimistic about what is to come."[5]

Jeff said, "I was searching for an effective diet plan for years but I was not able to get something interesting. Maybe, my standards were high...I used different diet plans and lost some pounds but I was not satisfied until I started using intermittent fasting and keto diet. It is the single diet that helped me lose weight like crazy."[6]

Elizabeth said, "Intermittent fasting 16:8 and 24 hours for 11 days result. It is amazing from 60kg-56kg-54kg.

The struggle is real but it is all worth it. I started with 24-hour fasting for 2 days where you only drink lots of water and no food intake. From 6 am to 6 am the following day. After 24 hour fasting, I only fast starting 9 pm until 12 pm and the remaining 1 pm to 8 pm is allotted for eating. I only eat food for the entire 8 hours."

Alex said, "I was one of those kids who could eat anything they like and still be skinny (I just grew taller instead, finally reaching 6' 4"). I was also into many sports (swimming, tennis, football). In my 20s, I cycled to work every day (over 100 miles a week), which meant putting on weight was still never an issue for me. I was used to eating what I liked and as much as I liked and still being slim, but in my 30s when my son was born, I found I was too tired to cycle in to work, I would eat sugary snacks just to pep me up for the afternoon (which of course just meant I crashed an hour later and turned to more high sugar snacks...). I slowly put on weight but then took action (no unhealthy snacking at work) and slowly lost some of it again; until, that is, my daughter was born. Again, the sleepless nights with a baby caused a bad diet, eating to stay awake at work, too tired and zero energy, and no free time to exercise. I gained several kgs. I had always been between 85 kgs and 88 kgs (187-195 lbs) but I had gone up to 93 kgs (205 lbs). Not massive, but I felt I had no control. My thighs started rubbing together as I walked: o (. I thought there was no way 'back.' I had never been on a diet in my life and everything I had heard told me that "diets don't work!" You end up weighing more. People told me that weight gain is what happens as you get older, as your metabolism slows you get the middle age spread, that's life...but that's not how I see myself, and that's not how I want to be. But what could I do?

I have a biology degree so I began to read about the biomechanics of weight loss. I read about how hard it is and why people can't stick to diets - I read lots about metabolism and sugar, ketogenic diets, and then about insulin resistance and fasting... I watched documentaries and YouTube videos, which then led me to videos about fasting and the benefits. That's when I came across intermittent fasting; I could still eat for 8 hours a day and lose weight, build muscle, heal my body, and stop the all-day sugar rollercoaster. It seemed too good to be true! I started slowly, just missing breakfast and having black coffee (Yuk!!), then having lunch at 12 and eating normally, with dinner to finish at 8 pm. In the first couple of months I had hard days and easy days but the more I did the clean fast the easier it got (and the more I learned to love black coffee).

I eat two meals a day (TMAD), usually in an 8-hour window, and sometimes as low as 5 hours. Getting the feeling of being in ketosis and knowing I am burning fat, knowing I am in control of my weight, and knowing that I am going to be eating a large satisfying meal later all felt great. I eat so well: bread, beer, pizza, chocolate, ice-cream, hamburgers, steaks, cheese, pasta, bacon! But the longer I did IF, the smaller the quantity of food I wanted, and the healthier foods seemed so much more appealing. I am now 1.5 years in, doing IF every day (well most days). I am leaner now than I have ever been in my adult life (82kg) I am in control and I love this way of eating. It's so simple and easy to apply and I even love my black coffee. I have signed up for a triathlon this August, and I am learning about being a fat adapted athlete. I am looking forward to getting older, feasting on what I want and staying in great shape with ease. It's all so simple: Delay, don't deny!"[7]

Sheila said, "It's been 4 years in the making, with a lifetime to go! I refuse to allow food to control me, obesity to paralyze me, and fear of success to stagnate me. God has placed too much purpose in me to not walk it out. Intermittent fasting saved me."

Sharon said, "I did it!!!! Today marks my 365th day of IF and the first time in my life I've had the willpower to focus on my own health and happiness.

I'm 5'9" and always been "big boned" with an obese/overweight BMI. My highest weight was 192 lbs in October 2016 and I've lost less than 20 lbs since starting IF a year ago. I've always weighed "a lot," but that doesn't make it any easier to still have a BMI in the overweight range despite my commitment to clean fasting since day 1. For many, that small amount of loss would be a reason to quit.

I've spent most of my adult life in a size 12/14 weighing a little more than I do now, give or take. I started IF wearing size 10 jeans. This past summer I bought all new clothes in a size 8. Now they are all too big. I had to buy smaller underwear for the first time in my adult life. Large t-shirts are too big on me for the first time in my adult life. That string bikini I bought as a joke...well, it's too big. I've run several races over the past few years and all my running shorts/shirts are too big. I'm just about ready to commit to size 6 jeans...but not yet. I'm no longer the girl who is "large" everything. I weigh less than what is on my driver's license...and we all know that was a lie from the start. I am no longer the "biggest" person when in a group of people. If you have been this person without fail, you know how painful that is. IF has healed some of the autoimmune aspects of my hypothyroidism. I really do look younger! THIS is why we don't quit. THIS is why we trust the process.

I truly eat whatever I want during my window. I am REALLY good at delaying, knowing I don't have to deny. During the work week, I pretty much stick to OMAD. During the weekends, I have more of a window. We went on vacation this summer where I stuck to my window and had no weight gain. We went to Disney for a week where I stuck to an extended window and had no weight gain. This holiday season was the most relaxed I've been this whole year and the couple of pounds I gained (and will lose by the end of the week) were totally worth it. This flexibility and not restricting what I eat has been what helped me be successful. I'm sure I could lose more weight with more restrictions, but I can promise you I would have quit a long time ago. Besides, people don't see my scale but they certainly see my figure. If only my face would get with the program and slim on up...

My food preferences have definitely been the biggest change since starting IF. I'm not opposed to cake and sweets but I'm not as dependent on sugar as I once was. I used to NEED something sweet after eating or I would get shaky. I struggled with hypoglycemia on a regular basis...but not once in the last 365 days, even when donating blood. I crave veggies and quality proteins. I started eating/craving real, quality cheeses for the first time in my life. The thought of wasting my one meal on fast food, boxed meals, or cheap sandwiches hurts my soul. When I do want sweets, I gravitate toward a specific taste rather than anything and everything in the pantry. Poor Little Debbie is lost without me. Despite trying everything, I haven't been able to adapt to black coffee so I open my window every day with a cup of sweet, creamy coffee as my own little "high five" for sticking with it.

I know this is long, but I hope this helps someone else stay the course. I've watched my mom diet since the day I was born. I grew up never knowing what full-fat salad dressings and non-diet sodas tasted like. I never understood why she couldn't love herself and see her own beauty in the same way I loved her and thought she was beautiful. Then I became a mom and those little punks did to my body what I did to hers. It became very hard to feel worthy or lovable. I dabbled in Weight Watchers, counted calories once, and took ONE diet pill (no thanks) but could never commit because I knew they didn't work. I'd watched my mom lose and gain and lose and gain my whole childhood. She has the willpower of steel and I knew I wouldn't be able to measure up. But this...THIS WORKS. Maybe I haven't lost a lot of weight, but I have healed a very broken body and have patched up a much-damaged soul. This was for me. I can say, without a doubt, IF has become and will remain my lifestyle."[8]

Brown said, "A lot of people ask me what workouts will help with belly fat and the answer is none. There is no specific workout that will target belly fat. Abdominal workouts are great for building muscle but fat loss comes in the form of creating a caloric budgeting or doing cardio. In order to have your abs muscles show, you must build the muscles while also shedding the fat that is covering them. Intermittent fasting rocks!"

Nicole said, "I lost 25 pounds in like 4 months. But that was with a lot of slip-ups. Like I had planned on fasting one day, and I would get invited to an office party or my roommates' parents for dinner. It is very hard for me to turn down food when someone makes it for me. But I still lost weight. Intermittent fasting really saved my life because I do not know how I could have survived."

Theusan said, "I have been on Intermittent fasting for a month or so, and have lost 2, maybe 3 pounds? I am pretty low BF already, so every pound is a bit of a battle, but I have really come to enjoy the rhythm of it, and I will probably still intermittent fasting at maintenance and maybe even through my bulk this winter. Really it just helps me enjoy my meals more and think about food less."

Gabriella said, "I've never been able to do the normal diets - eating disorder since I was a teen (binge/purge), thinking that was a great way to lose weight. For me, there were good foods and bad foods. If I ate the good ones, I was ok. If I ate anything I considered bad, I felt this overwhelming urge to get rid of it. The weight kept going up - every 5 pounds I gained, I wished I was where I'd been 5 pounds ago. I had short periods of lower weight while doing Community Theatre, nightly walking my dog and jazzercise.

I actually visited friend years ago and saw she'd lost weight - she said she ate dinner only, whatever she wanted. At the time, that just sounded crazy to me and I dismissed it - wish I'd paid better attention.[9]

I cleaned up my diet while doing some research on living on a food-stamp budget. Less eating out, more eating at home. Joined a co-op and started getting lots of fruit and vegetables to play with.

In the spring of 2015, I ran my first ever 5k and at the pre-race pasta party, Team World Vision was there and said they could take me from 5k to marathon in time for the Chicago marathon in October.

For whatever reason, I believed them and signed up. I spent that summer training, along with some weight training to strengthen my legs. I thought all that running would HAVE to help me lose weight. I finished that marathon, very slowly. I only lost 10 pounds, which went right back on when I quit running.

In late 2016, I found IF (intermittent fasting) and OMAD (one meal a day). I remembered that friend I'd visited. I started in January 2017 at a weight of 172, wearing mostly size 14s.

I saw absolutely no loss per the scale for at least 3 weeks, but my belly was going away and clothes were fitting looser. I did a 72 hour fast and dropped 5 pounds, sat there for a while; another long fast with a drop, and sat there - but then my body seemed to start to learn what to do.

I generally use a 4-hour eating window but have had some longer ones when something comes up. I don't restrict because that would make me obsess. No journaling, because that would also make me crazy.

It's now September 2017. I wobble between 146 and 148, but my body looks completely different. I'm wearing anywhere from 4s to 8s in clothes. I'm sleeping well, my skin looks better, and I have tons of energy. I had a physical recently and the doctor said all my lab tests look great - my HDL was so high it offset my high LDL.

IF and OMAD gave me back my life, a life with confidence and food freedom."[10]

Chapter Two: Why Intermittent Fasting Works

It is very obvious and vividly clear that intermittent fasting is a reviving lifestyle and one of the most effective ways for weight loss, staying healthy and fit, and a whole lot of other benefits associated within.

In its simplest form, intermittent fasting is a fitness trend of eating where you put your body system through various cycles of abstaining and intentionally not eating or consuming food for a number of assigned and specified hours. Starters commonly begin with a 12-hour cycle where they permit themselves to consume or eat food from 8am to 8pm, and then they would proceed into fasting mode where they do not eat or consume any food of all manner from 8pm to 8am.

The act of intermittent fasting has received global popularity due to the enormous number of research and studies that have ascertained over time the wonderful benefits to be gained. Alongside being a very effective treatment for overweight and obesity, intermittent fasting has proven to increase and make better some health-related factors and age-associated loss of tissue function. In order for you to get a better understanding on how and why making ourselves go through such a fasting timetable is very effective for a longer lifespan and massive weight loss, I have decided to make mention of interviews that have been done with experts in the field.

According to a Harvard trained physician who is also the author of The Paleovedic Diet, Dr. Akil Palanisamy, "*intermittent fasting works primarily via three mechanisms. The primary one is hormone balance. It boosts growth hormone levels and normalizes metabolic hormones like insulin, leptin, and ghrelin. In men, it is also believed to raise testosterone. The second is fat burning. It is one of the most effective techniques for boosting metabolism and promoting the breakdown of adipose tissue. Third, it promotes autophagy, which is the process by which cells break down tox-*

ins and debris. This helps regenerate cells and has an anti-aging effect as well."[11]

The founder of Ancient Nutrition and DrAxe.com, Dr. Josh Axe, explains further in his website that, *"the extensive research on the concept of intermittent fasting suggests it functions in two different ways to improve various facets of health. First, intermittent fasting results in lowered levels of oxidative stress to cells throughout the body. This is believed to be the mechanism behind IF's protection of the heart and brain particular, as well as its impact on lifespan."* On another note, Dr. Axe continues that, *"practicing IF improves your body's ability to deal with stress at a cellular level. Intermittent fasting activates cellular stress response pathways similar to very mild stressors, acting as mild stimulants for your body's stress response. As this occurs consistently, your body is slowly reinforced against cellular stress and is then less susceptible to cellular aging and disease development."*[12]

It is very important to note that engaging in intermittent fasting alone won't be as effective. In order to take full advantage of the effectiveness and benefits of intermittent fasting, Dr. Chad Walding, co-founder of NativePath and The Paleo Secret, and a holistic health coach, has once said that nutrition also plays a key role in intermittent fasting. He cautions that one should not have the false belief that *"you can binge on processed, high-sugar foods and then fast make up for it. There still is no silver bullet to sustainable weight loss and holistic health. Eating an anti-inflammatory diet full of a variety of vegetables and fruits, lean proteins, and quality fats are the dietary baseline for optimal health. From there, individuals need to find what works with their own unique biological blueprint."*[13]

This declares that we should not just eat and hope to change the wrong with fasting. Good nutrition works hand in hand with intermittent fasting. You should not consume too many calories or take in high sugar edibles and hope that your fasting will redeem it.

That is a blunt NO because the outcome of such fasting will not be vivid and encouraging. So we are encouraged to also participate in a good nutritional diet (like a ketogenic diet) while engaging in intermittent fasting and there would be results that would be self-encouraging and would push to you to continue in the lifestyle.

Another view into why intermittent fasting works is that the excess weight that you want to shed in your body is stored up energy which was turned into fat. It is through the consumption of calories that energy is found, and calories are gotten from the food we eat. So you see that intermittent fasting finds a way for you to minimize the number of mind-blowing calories you eat by abstaining from food for a period of time.

During this period of not consuming calories, the body system would have no option but to use the stored energy, that is, fat, in order to go on with the day to day activities you engage in. This is a great medium of reducing the excess fat gotten from excess calories and use it for energy of the body. Therefore, no excess energy is stored up and that means no excess fat. This can be mind-blowing sometimes but it is simply one of the various ways by which intermittent fasting works in your body.

After a long series of intermittent fasting, as long as you do not eat too much or extravagantly, intermittent fasting will really help you reduce excess weight and belly fat.

Studies have shown that intermittent fasting, if properly followed, can be a very useful and powerful tool in weight loss. A review study carried out in 2014 has found out that this eating pattern [intermittent fasting] can cause 3-8% weight loss over a period of 3-24 weeks, which is quite a significant amount when compared to most weight loss studies.

This same study has revealed that people also tend to lose 4-7% of their waist circumference; this indicates a significant loss of dangerous and harmful belly fat which builds up around your organs and causes disease. Another study has shown that intermittent fasting causes less muscle loss than the more standard method of continuous calorie restriction schemes.

Myths/Misconceptions Regarding Intermittent Fasting

There are a lot for misconceptions regarding intermittent fasting; most of these misconceptions are laughable due to their ingenuity and lack of concrete proof to back them up. I would separate the truth from fiction and ingenuity.

Intermittent fasting has received a lot of recognition from experts and enthusiasts over the years following its efficacy. This has led to a few myths and misconceptions surrounding what intermittent fasting actually dictate.

It is not an astonishing fact that the number of people who are against the intermittent fasting lifestyle is mind-blowing proportional to the people who diligently follow its dictates. There is a clear logic to this, which means there is some iota of effectiveness and sound reasoning following the intermittent fasting lifestyle's course.

Instead of praising and emphasizing the benefits of intermittent fasting, I will look at some of the unfounded myths and claims about the devastating advantage of intermittent fasting and provide a sound rebuttal to the claim that it is a wrong and unhealthy way of living.

First, it is widely believed by some people that your metabolism will increase if you eat frequently. It is quite laughable that this belief is floating around the internet. *"Eat many, small meals to stoke the metabolic flame."*

Many people have the belief that eating more meals leads to a high chance of increasing your metabolic rate, in order for your body to burn more calories overall.

I would not dispute the fact that the human body expends a certain amount of energy in digesting and using the nutrients that are in a meal. This is known as the thermic effect of food and it amounts to about 20-30% of calories for protein, 5-10% carbohydrate, 3% for fat.

Averagely, the thermic effect of food ranges up to around 10% of the total calorie intake. The main contention of this is the total number of calories that are consumed, not the number of meals that are eaten. For example, eating ten 600 calorie meals still has the same effect as eating six 1000 calories meals. It is still the same amount, which is 10%, it is still 600 calories in both cases. This is supported by various studies regarding feeding in humans, showing that decreasing or increasing of meal frequency has no effect on the total calories burned. Your total calorie intake is what matters.

It is the belief of some people that snacking and eating often and frequently is very good for the health. It is not natural for the human body to be in a constant state of being fed. When we were evolving, there were times we had to be in a state of scarcity periodically.

It has been proven that intermittent fasting induces a cellular repair process called autophagy, whereby the cells use old proteins for the purpose of energy. This process helps against many diseases like Alzheimer's disease and it has even been said to reduce the chances of cancer.

In an interview, Dr. Chaldwin said, "*The truth is that fasting from time to time has all sort of benefits for metabolic health. There are some studies that have shown that snacking, and eating very often, can have negative effects on health and raise your risk of disease.*"

A study found out that, with high-calorie intake included, a diet with more frequent meals causes a higher and greater increase in liver fat, indicating that snacking may raise the risk of fatty liver disease. Also, it has been revealed that people that eat more often have a higher risk of having colorectal cancer. It is a misconception that snacking is good for the health. Various studies show that snacking is quite harmful and some other studies show that engaging in intermittent fasting from time to time has major health benefits.

A very common and widespread allegation about intermittent fasting is that it puts the body in a mode of starvation. Can this be said to be true? According to the allegation, the act of not eating [intermittent fasting] makes the body think it is starving; therefore it shuts down its metabolism and prevents you from burning calories.

It is quite true that long-term weight loss can actually reduce the number of calories an individual burns. But this generally happens with weight loss, no matter which method you use. There is no factual evidence that pinpoints that it is only intermittent fasting it happens to because this is common with other weight loss strategies. As a matter of fact, it has been proven that intermittent fasting increases the rate of metabolism. This is due to a drastic rise in blood levels of norepinephrine, which instructs the fat cells to break down body fat and also stimulate metabolism.

It has been said that intermittent fasting is not good for people with diabetes. The belief that we need to consume food constantly in order to maintain your blood sugar level is an intermittent fasting myth that pervades the society as a whole.

A study has shown that through intermittent fasting, there has been stabilization in the blood sugar of partakers after having dinner. In a group of type 2 diabetics, there has been improved weight loss, and there have also been improved blood sugar levels.

In fact, long fasting has even been said to be able to restore insulin sensitivity in those suffering from type 2 diabetes. Also following a ketogenic diet routine judiciously has been also proven to restore insulin sensitivity as well because the better our insulin sensitivity, the less insulin our body will have to produce and this will lead to less inflammation in our body system.

This is of utmost importance because it reduces the risk of kidney failure and heart disease in people that are suffering from diabetes.

Another great thing is that for individuals that are suffering from diabetes type 1 and cannot produce their own insulin, it is very important to closely monitor blood sugar to do this right. So you see that not only has this belief been disproved, it has also been made known that intermittent fasting is very useful to people that are suffering from diabetes.

I came across a write up on a particular day that claims intermittent fasting causes muscle loss and I decided to address the issue. This is one of the myths of intermittent fasting and it is mostly originating from the fitness world. It is a misconception. It is true that the body will proceed into creating energy from the proteins in the muscles during the period of elongated calorie restriction; this is unlikely to happen during a daily intermittent fast.

As a matter of fact, a recent test showed that alternate day fasting for a period of 8 weeks stimulates fat loss on an average of 12 lbs while there is no vivid or significant loss or reduction in the muscle mass. The good news is that you can actually lose weight and also gain muscle at the same time while engaging in intermittent fasting. How is that possible? Just optimize your calorie and protein intake within your eating window. With intermittent fasting, you can still gain more muscles.

It is also believed that the brain will not get enough fuel in order to carry out activities. This is one of the common myths of intermittent fasting but it will be rebutted. It is a common belief among people that without food the brain cannot function properly. I remember when I was in elementary school, my mom would always tell me in the morning while preparing to go to school that if I do not eat, my brain would not function properly in school. Is this really true?

It has been proven not to be true. The claim says that if you are fasting, your brain cannot function properly and you will lose concentration and your memory. Not exactly. The brain does need glucose to operate. If you do not eat every few hours, your brain will not stop functioning. Even during a prolonged fast, the body can still produce what the brain will function from.

We have now examined various claims, myths and misconceptions regarding the act of intermittent fasting, which I hope have been rebutted and have been made vividly clear.

Chapter Three: What Do We Mean By Ketogenic Diet?

I know this might not really be the first time you are seeing this word, "*ketogenic*."

To understand deeply what lies beneath the word, we need to understand certain terms.

What is a diet? In the world of nutrition, a diet can be referred to as the summation of food that is consumed by a person or any other organism. This word often insinuates the use of a peculiar intake of nutrition for the purpose of health or weight management.

No disputing the fact that we humans can be described as omnivorous creatures. Each person and individual culture holds in high esteem some food preference and some food taboos. This can be due to some personal reasons and convictions or personal taste and ethics. These individual choices may be very healthy while some can be less healthy.

What is a ketogenic diet? A ketogenic diet is high fat, low carbohydrate, and adequate protein diet that in the world of medicine, was used to treat refractory epilepsy in children.

This diet urges the body to burn fats rather than burning carbohydrates contained in food which is converted to glucose, and it is then transferred around the human body, having the sole purpose of fuelling the brain, cells and all. However, if the diet has very little carbohydrates, the liver converts the fats into fatty acids and ketone bodies.

These ketone bodies pass into the brain and they replace the glucose as an energy source. A state in the human body whereby there is an elevated level of ketones in the blood is known as ketosis and this drastically reduces the rate of epileptic seizures.

Ketosis is a natural state for the human body when it is almost totally fuelled by fat. This is normal during fasting or when you are on a strict low carbohydrate diet which is also known as a ketogenic diet.

When you are experiencing ketosis, there are a lot of benefits and advantages which are related to the reduction in weight mass, performance, and health.

The word "*keto*" in ketosis is derived from "*ketones*," and as I have said earlier, ketones are from the conversion of fats and it also means small fuel molecules that are in the body.

It is an alternative fuel and energy source for the body, produced from the fats we eat and it is most significantly used when the glucose in our body is very short in supply.

These ketones are produced when you eat a very low carbohydrate diet [carbs are the main source of glucose] and a moderate amount of proteins because excess protein can also be converted to blood sugar.

This state of ketosis is very beneficial; a certain way of entering this state is through a ketogenic diet.

During the process of the ketogenic diet, the body is not supplied enough blood sugar from carbohydrate and proteins.

This will force the liver to convert the fat to fatty acids and ketones, which fuels the brain and leads to a state of ketosis.

During this state, the body switches its entire energy supply into fat and completely burns it which will lead to massive fat burn and weight loss, and the level of fat storing hormone insulin also reduces.

Studies have shown that this is very great for weight loss. You can ask that, how do I get into this ketosis? To get into ketosis, you need a low level of the fat storing hormone insulin and this can be achieved by engaging in a ketogenic diet and also adding intermittent fasting. The ketogenic diet has been proven by research and studies to treat epilepsy, acne, and it also helps in weight loss and controlling blood sugar.

The Historical Development Of Ketogenic Diet

The history of the ketogenic diet can be dated to the 1920s and 1930s. The ketogenic diet became widely known as a form of therapy for epilepsy. The ketogenic diet was developed to provide an alternative to non-mainstream fasting which has demonstrated its success as an effective epilepsy therapy. However, the ketogenic diet was later abandoned due to the invention of anticonvulsant therapies. Although, it was proven that the medication could control most cases of epilepsy, they still failed to control about 20-30% of epileptic cases especially in cases of small children and the ketogenic diet was reintroduced as a way of managing the condition.

It was in 1921 that an endocrinologist Rollin Woodyatt observed and made note that three water-soluble compounds, acetone, acetoacetate and beta hydroxybutyrate which are called ketone bodies were produced by the liver as a result of starvation or if they followed a diet which is rich in fats and low in carbohydrates.

Russell Wilder from the Mayo Clinic called this the ketogenic diet and started using it as a treatment of epilepsy in 1921.

Extended researches that were carried out in the 1960s showed that more ketones are produced by medium chain triglycerides per unit of energy because they were transferred quickly to the liver.

In 1971, Peter Huttenlocher came out with a ketogenic diet whereby 60% of its calories were derived from medium chain triglycerides oil and more carbohydrates and protein be added compared with the original ketogenic diet. This insinuates that meals could be prepared more enjoyably by the parents for their children that have epilepsy. Many hospitals adopted the MCT diet in place of the original ketogenic diet, while some of them used the combination of the two.

The ketogenic diet received national media limelight in the United States in October 1994, when the NBC's program made mention of the case of Charlie Abrahams. The two-year-old suffered severely from epilepsy, which remained uncontrolled by the mainstream and alternative therapies.

His father Jim Abrahams found a reference to the ketogenic diet in an epilepsy guide and took Charlie to John M. Freeman at Johns Hopkins Hospital, where the therapy was continually offered. Charlie's epilepsy was drastically controlled under the ketogenic diet and his developmental progress continued.

This greatly inspired Abrahams to create the Charlie foundation in order to improve the ketogenic diet and fund research.

There was a scientific explosion that pointed interest in the ketogenic diet. In 1997, Abrahams produced a movie, in which a young boy who was suffering from epilepsy was successfully treated by the ketogenic diet. By 2007, the ketogenic diet was made available from around 75 centers in 45 countries. The ketogenic diet was also praised and is under investigation for treating other disorders aside from epilepsy.

Testimonies Acknowledging The Efficacy Of The Ketogenic Diet

As I mentioned earlier in the historical development of the ketogenic diet, I made mention of Charlie Abrahams whose success story triggered the distribution of knowledge and the enlightenment of people to know the effectiveness of the ketogenic diet.

Many people have had several testimonies to the value and how important the ketogenic diet is. I have come across a lot of testimonies that are heart-melting, breathtaking, and make me want to take a megaphone and testify to the efficacy of the ketogenic diet around the world. In this segment, the testimonies of such people would be shared.

These testimonies are taken from various websites and will be referenced as footnotes, and also at the end of the book.

Abigail said, "*My 31-day transformation! The last few months of 2017 were rough for me. With so many life changes happening, I found myself at the corner of mental and physical exhaustion. Bottling so many inside, I let my stress take the best of me. I started to neglect my health in ways I have not done in years. I desperately needed positive change. I desperately needed myself back...*

I talk about the horrible side effects that happened to me during those 3 months of neglect and how keto diet has saved me from totally regretting how I have turned. It was very hard at first because I have already gotten used to the type of food I used to eat."[14]

A fit mom said, *"17.5 inches and I lost 23 pounds!!!*

Today is a big, big deal for me.

I am celebrating 60 days of keto and I have lost and gained so many things!

What I have lost on keto

- 23 pounds
- 2.25 inches on arms
- 3 inches on waist
- 5.5 inches on hips
- 3.5 inches on pooch
- 1.75 inches on each thigh
- 1.5 inches on each calf.

You guys, I lost 23 pounds and more than 17.5 inches in only 60 days in ketosis

Because of having surgery only a couple of weeks into my 60-day goal, I was not even able to work out much, and so I am just now getting back into the swing of power lifting again, so almost all of this is by diet alone.

I did not count calories; I only counted my carb and stayed below 40 net carbs every day.

So what comes next?

Well first, new swimsuits. Mine are falling off, and I can see baby abs coming through, so hello two piece!

I am also sticking with keto a bit longer, because my friend is still on to lose weight for the military but after that I am going to be doing modified keto where I consume about 25 g of carbs 30 minutes before my workout for a couple of months, and then gauge if I am still losing fat and gaining muscle.

My body is an experiment right now, but worst case scenario I will be unhappy with adding in more carbs and will go back to keto."[15]

Linda said, "Hi there, my name is Linda; I have lost just over 60lbs using keto diet, started in early November, I am getting married in 2019, and looking to be my best self! My goal is to lose 100-110lbs total."

Natalie said, "I consumed gluten here and there...thank God I got tested for food sensitivities or I would be in poor health still. Nothing against the vegan diet, but everyone's body is different, People have had success with veganism and people who are insulin resistant haven't. So glad I found Keto, it has saved my life."[16]

A mom from Texas said, "Gosh I remember the feelings I had before I started keto...feelings of fear, feelings of being discouraged or letting myself down again...what if I fail at this like I have with every other thing I have tried for the past 12 years. Looking back a year ago on Mother's Day reflecting where I was then to where I am now not just my weight loss but also my mental state at the time. Things were better, but I was nowhere near where I am now. The weight loss and drastically changing my eating habits have all contributed and I am so thankful I made myself show up every day. So, what if? What if I never gave myself the chance? I preach believing in yourself a lot because you are the only one who can push yourself to make the change. Do not let the ifs hold you back. Believe in YOU. Show up for YOU. Tiptoe if you must but if it is something you want so bad... every day wake up and TAKE THAT STEP! IT IS WORTH IT. All thanks to KETO.[17]

A keto wife said, "I have been in keto for 42 days now! I have never been so happy with a diet in my life. I have lost 26 pounds, keto really saved my life. I am encouraged to keep going as I want to achieve my desired goal. Along with diet I also exercise about 3 days a week to keep a healthy life. Keto saved me."[18]

A transformed woman said, "I started my keto diet late September and I am currently still dieting. I lost 35lbs by the beginning of March. I had my daughter in January 2017. After caring for my new family, I forgot to care about myself. I forgot to keep myself healthy and happy. The keto diet and regular exercise have made me into the healthy mom and wife and family and I deserve."[19]

Becky said, "Oh, what a difference a year makes! Keto has worked wonders for my body. Last year I weighed about 13 lbs heavier and I was running or doing cardio every day but eating tons of carbs. Now I still work out every day, but function high-fat fat diet."

Sugar said, "Happy translation Tuesday. I can honestly say a year ago, I never would have imagined surpassing my goal of a 50 lbs weight loss, but here I am 75 lbs lighter and feeling better than ever! The girl I was before was ashamed of her body and would cover it up to make sure no one would see it. The new girl I am now is confident, empowered, and strong! I feel so lucky to have a great support system around me and thank all of you who have reached out for advice or sent kind words. Keep calm and Keto on, friends.

In four days, it will be 6 months I have been on my weight loss journey with the help of keto, 31 lbs down. This has been a journey but I love every moment of it. It is not over yet."

Amy said, "I have been asked a lot about keto, and if I think it really works. As of today...I have lost almost 40 pounds, have a ton of energy and I am seeing a difference with my memory. This is not a diet; it is a way of life. If I can eat cheese and lose weight...count me in."[20]

Nicole wrote, "I used to be severely overweight for a period of my life. Some people have known me a long time and they have seen my progress, but some only know me now and do not know what I used to be. There are a few years of my life with zero to few pictures of me because I hated the way I looked. After getting out of a toxic relationship when I ate my feelings out of depression, I was able to lose a little bit on my own by focusing on me getting back into activities I loved which were musical theatre and overall being happy again. But I was still overweight and sort of hit a plateau, so I gave up on trying because nothing seemed to be working. It was not until October of 2016 that I learned about ketogenic lifestyle and started that way of eating and was able to lose 10 pounds in 2 months, just from making better food choices. In January of 2017, I began a fitness regime, going to the gym about 4-5 days a week doing a mix of weight lifting and cardio. My plan was to hit my goal weight within one year. To be honest, I did not think I was going to do it but told myself I would be happy if I got close. It has been one year since I did my first workout on my own and I am so excited to say that I did it...I hit my goal weight!!! From June 2015 to now, I have lost 76 pounds and I am a happier, healthier, and stronger version of myself than I ever was before. It is not just about the number and how I look, but I have learned that I need to take care of my body from the inside out for health reasons too. I now have more energy and I feel absolutely amazing. I finally feel like the version of myself that I always envisioned in my head. This has been a long and hard journey and there were times I thought I might give up. I am sharing this not out of vanity, but because I am just so happy that I want people to know that you can do whatever you set your mind to!!"[21]

Salem wrote, "I did not have a problem with losing weight. The problems were with other diets that I had tried before did not account for a long-term result so I ended up always gaining back the weight that I lost. I was depressed with the way I looked, had no interest or energy, my mood was erratic. I was facing new psychological problems with phobias. I needed a solution; I wanted to turn to drugs.

I was glad and happy that I found the ketogenic diet and I was extremely doubtful and thought it was just another fad diet. I started and I was just amazed, not just the weight loss, but my mood, my emotions, my energy all came back. I was feeling as energetic and youthful as a teenager. Keto is not a diet; it is a way of life. Thank you, Keto, for how you have saved me."[22]

Vincent wrote, "Just before last summer my doctor told me I had to lose weight, again. At that time I was 94 kg. My non-alcoholic fatty liver disease had returned. It had improved by losing weight the last time. But after slimming once again I regained the lost weight and the fatty liver came back. My iron was out of limits. The doctor gave me a summary table of the calories from different foods. The message I got was that I should reduce the amount of calories that I was eating. It is a nice doctor, but he has no idea about nutrition, obviously. Anyway, I started to eat less again. I also increased the amount of exercise I was doing, spending at least half an hour every day on the exercise bike. Instinctively, I eliminated bread and pasta from my diet and I started eating very little, about 1200 calories per day. I was often hungry, but I have willpower. I used a ketogenic diet to control what I was eating. I began to see tremendous changes, changes that have not happened in a long time. All thanks to the keto diet."

Vivian said during an interview, "Here is one that I do not know if you have heard of before with ketogenic lifestyle, my warts of many years are falling off. Literally, I am thrilled. I have a few more that are starting to change and will apparently be leaving soon. I have only been doing the ketogenic diet for about 7 weeks now: I have lost 8 lbs easily. It just seemed to melt off into the 2nd/3rd week. I feel more grounded and centered, not flighty and spacey, foggy-headed. I am more peaceful and calm. My poops are great now. This is an important part, lady. I used to have major digestive issues and constipation but in my second and third week, everything changed. My belly bloat was gone. I have always had blood sugar issues since a child and now, with the way I am eating, I do not have it. I am still learning more through this journey and I am pleased. I highly recommend it to anyone. I have had people asking what I am doing. I am radiant and healthy looking than ever. I started telling them about keto. All thanks to keto."[23]

Katie also wrote that "I have been on keto since July of this year:

- 18 pounds lost
- 4 inches lost off my waist, 4 inches lost off my hips
- Down three sizes
- Down 3.5 percentage points in body fat
- Shaved a minute off of my mile time
- No longer pre-diabetic
- Periods regular for the first time in my life
- Not a single migraine since starting
- My skin looks ten years younger
- No more issues with sugar blood spikes and crashes, which has gone a long way in helping manage my depressions without medications
- Increased energy and mental clarity[24]

Christine who has gone through a total transformation wrote and said, "I never in a million years thought that I would share my story, but after a very emotional weekend looking at one of my year old picture and lots of encouragement.

That picture is one year apart from a very unhealthy, metabolically sick 49-year-old transformed to a healthy, energetic 50-year-old. I am completely blown away by the changes.

In October 2016, I had been on a quitting sugar journey for a few months and had successfully given up the white, sweet stuff. Desserts, cookies, and packaged foods were no longer part of my diet but were resulting in a very slow weight loss. I started this journey to lose weight, and to reverse metabolic syndrome, fatty liver, insulin resistance, and if I was very lucky, sleep apnoea.

I was complaining about the slow loss to a friend and she asked me if I was familiar with ketogenic fasting. I had never heard of the keto way of eating. On that day, January 13, 2017, I came home and secured the internet for information. January 13, 2017, was the last day I ate potatoes, bread, and pasta. Those were the final high carbohydrate foods that I kicked to the curb and as a result, I had excellent results with weight loss. Because I had already quit sugar, there was little difficulty or withdrawal. I am pretty sure I entered ketosis state within a week of ditching those high starchy carbohydrates.

Nine months on the ketogenic and intermittent fasting journey, I have dropped over 80lbs and I am so very close to a healthy weight. I have also lost: daily headaches, monthly migraines, cystic acne, ovarian cysts, lethargic afternoons and evenings, joint pain, inflammation, and best of all, sleep apnoea. I no longer have to use a CPAP machine (confirmed with another sleep test that my obstructive sleep apnoea is gone). I have gained: a renewed joy for life, more energy than I know what to do with, a new appreciation for real food and cooking, shopping in regular size shops, improved self-esteem!

Turning fifty has been the best thing that has ever happened to me because it really lit a fire in caring for my personal health. My biggest challenge was letting go of potato chips but repeating a question to myself as to what those would do to my insulin response, I was able to break that addiction and have no desire for those foods that obviously make me sick.

My biggest regret is not knowing about this way of life earlier, but I truly believe God's hand was in this journey with me every step of the way making it easy to adopt this new lifestyle to stick with it 100%. I am so very grateful for real food and ketogenic diet; it has truly given me the gift of life to enjoy with my family and friends for many years to come. Here is to the next 50 years! Thanks to keto diet!!!"

Six months ago, I had my annual visit with my primary care provider of twenty years. My knees hurt, and I was 30 pounds (14 kg) overweight, confirmed by my BMI. My cholesterol was 282 mg/dl, my "bad" cholesterol was high, my "good" cholesterol and triglycerides could have been better, but my calculated VLDL was OK.[25]

Beatrice said, "For the knee pain, my PCP added "osteoarthritis" to my problem list. For the elevated cholesterol, she recommended exercise and a low-fat diet, a trope which she has sung to me for two decades.

"Fine," I thought. "But my knee pain is the problem that is bothering me the most. It is not only limiting my ability to exercise, but it is limiting my daily activities. And you, knowing by my report that I am not ready to contemplate knee replacements, have essentially told me to 'live with it.'

It seemed to me that my first-line effort to deal with my knee pain should be weight loss. About a week after I saw my doctor, I stumbled across www.dietdoctor.com. I read the scientific studies regarding low-carbohydrate, high-fat diets on www.dietdoctor.com and in medical journals. I emailed my doctor and reiterated that what concerned me the most was my limited mobility due to my knee pain. I told her my plan: "I am going to try a ketogenic diet for six months and recheck my lipids at that time. If I lose weight, and my knees stop hurting, but my lipids get worse, I will take a stating." Her response: "Well, that is an interesting approach."

Six months into a low-carbohydrate, high-fat diet that probably doesn't quite make it to ketogenic most of the time, I have lost 28 pounds (13 kg). My BMI is normal. I lost 6″ (15 cm) around my waist, and I have gone down four pants sizes. Most importantly, my knee pain is much, much better. I checked my lipids at a free screening offered by a local pharmacy: My total cholesterol, triglycerides, and "bad" cholesterol were all DOWN from six months ago. My "good" cholesterol was UP. I feel great and feel wholly vindicated in my "interesting approach."

For me, a low-carbohydrate, high-fat diet has been easy to follow. I knew I couldn't face recording carbohydrates after decades of off-and-on meticulous food record-keeping that calorie in-calorie out dieting entails.

I like coffee, it does not give me heartburn or palpitations, and I have the leisure to sleep late and drink multiple cups in the morning. So, instead of breakfast, I enjoy two or three cups of coffee with heavy cream in the morning while I check my email, social media, plan my day, do my household chores, etc. At about 10 or 11, I am hungry enough to eat, so I'll have a "brunch" of bacon and eggs or smoked salmon or ham, and fresh mozzarella cheese with avocado and maybe some sliced tomato. By then I am tired of coffee, so for a beverage, I have water (still or sparkling) or a glass of unsweetened coconut milk. I am not hungry again until dinner, which I prepare using one of the www.dietdoctor.com recipes or a low-carbohydrate adaptation of one of our family favourites.

Dining out is relatively simple: I have grilled meat or fish and double vegetables instead of the offered starch plus vegetables. If the only option is burgers, I ask for one without the bun or remove the bun when the burger is served. At first, I had to ask the server to take away the table bread; now I just ignore it. I also make it a point to eat a zero-carbohydrate snack before I dine out so that the table bread is less tempting. I have never been much of an evening snack eater, but I do enjoy a glass or two of white wine in the evening. Lately, though, I enjoy that less (I have found that I feel its adverse effects much more now, and much more quickly) and will skip that in favour of sparkling water or homemade eggnog[1] (pasteurized eggs, heavy cream, water, and no sugar or artificial sweetener).

My current dilemma is what to do now that I have achieved my goals of weight loss and decreased knee pain. I am concerned that if I get even a little bit liberal with my carbohydrates, I will reactivate some triggers that will derail a sustained low-carbohydrate high-fat lifestyle. For now, I plan to continue eating as I have been for the past six months

---

1. https://www.dietdoctor.com/recipes/low-carb-eggnog

and reassess if my weight gets too low. That, for sure, would be a problem that would be a joy to tackle!"[26]

Rachael wrote, "Hi, this is my story, it's long but hey, I'm 62 years young. I am writing this story for myself, so I can be accountable to myself.

I can't even begin to tell you how many diets I have been on since elementary school.

I was a very sick kid until I was 5 when I got my tonsils out. My parents feed me milkshakes and ice cream most of the time. Well, let me tell you, once I was better, they gave me all the things I had missed! Both my parents were obese, and to top it off, we're Jewish, you know what that means. I had the typical Jewish grandmother who wants you to eat all the time or you'll starve. I became the fat kid in the family.

My parents divorced when I was 3, my mom was young and fed us what she could afford, which was potatoes, rice, and pasta. Need I say more? My mom lost her weight and didn't want me to go thru what she did as a child. I started with yo-yo dieting young.

My sisters didn't have a weight problem, so we always had junk food in our house (I became a closet eater). My mom would take me to doctors and they would always put me on a diet. I would always gain the weight back. By the time I was in high school I was probably 50 pounds (23 kg) overweight.

Believe it or not, when I was 21 there was an article in Cosmopolitan magazine called "Fasting the Ultimate Diet" and of course I had to try it. I fasted for 42 days while I was a cook on a fast food truck (first one off the assembly line, 43 years ago), and smoked two packs of cigarettes a day. I lost around 50 pounds (23 kg) and then got pregnant with my first son. So, I had to start eating and quit smoking ASAP. Well, you can imagine the outcome of that. Gained all the weight I lost back, plus an extra 35 pounds (16 kg). My excuse was I was eating for two, but when he was born, I only lost ten pounds (5 kg). I never lost the weight and got pregnant again with my second son. I gained

50 more pounds (23 kg) with him. So, between both of them, I gained 130 pounds (59 kg)!

When my second son was 10 months old, I was waiting to get on a program through the hospital called Medifast. It was a liquid diet that they monitored once a week with blood tests and weekly classes on food and nutrition. I went in for the initial tests, but the whole time my stomach was bothering me. When I got home, I was very sick with stabbing pains in my gut. I ended up going to the hospital and staying for a bunch of tests. They did exploratory surgery and I had pancreatitis. My whole system was poisoned, and the Doctor told me if I hadn't gone to the hospital when I did I probably would have died. I was in there for three weeks. For the first time in my life, they did not want me to lose any weight and to let my body heal for 6 months. My weight in the hospital was 297 lbs (134 kg).

I waited for six months and then started the Medifast program at the hospital. I lost 98 pounds (44 kg) in four months (not one bite of food, all liquid shakes.) Then I ate some BBQ chicken and the diet was over for me. I never could get back on the fast.

Then my sister got married and I was her Maid of Honor. I wore a gorgeous dress, and everyone thought I looked beautiful. Eight months later my sister died of a drug overdose. I was so crushed and mad, all I did was eat. I gained all my weight back, plus some.

For the next nine years, I went on many diets and would lose weight just to gain it back again. In 1991 I ended up in the hospital with a herniated disk in my neck. I had to have emergency surgery 5 days before Christmas. Because they had waited so long to operate, my left side was going numb down to my knee.

Then in 1992, I went through a divorce and lost 75 pounds (34 kg) and moved to Las Vegas to start over, and to be with all my family. My boys were 14 and 16 and they were a handful. As a single mom and a full-time manicurist, my life was busy, and I managed to get down to about 175 pounds (79 kg) and I felt pretty good about myself.

I was still heavy but felt I could live at this weight and be happy. I lived in Vegas for a year before I met my current husband. When we split for a while, I lost another 30 pounds (14 kg). Of course, that was starving me yet again. Which all of you know is the reason we gain the weight back. I couldn't continue this way of eating forever because I was hungry all the time. I am a nail tech, had a full clientele and no time to eat regular meals. We always had a ton of snacks around the beauty shop, so I would snack all day.

I got married and we moved back to Southern California and I couldn't get my nail license reinstated. I was home all day with nothing to do and ate out of boredom. In those three years of living there, I gained weight and then lost it, only to gain it back again. I never went above 198 pounds (90 kg). That is where I always started dieting; because I promised I would never get over 200 pounds (91 kg) again.

In 2002 we moved to Oregon where my husband was retired and wanted to have a small farm. I, on the other hand, decided to get my nail license and go back to work. I am a city girl who loves people and wanted to meet people in my new town. I figured the best way to meet people when you don't have kids growing up, is to go to work. I love doing nails.

Then in 2003, I had another major back surgery, on my lower back. So I tried to lose weight after that because my doctor said I had the back of an 80-year-old woman. So I went on another diet to give my back some relief. But, when you work in a beauty shop, there are always sweets and people bring in lots of baked goods. You guessed it – I ate. So for 12 years, the weight went up and down just about every two years. I have tried diets that were so crazy that now I can't even believe it.

Then in 2014, I was down to 155 pounds (70 lbs), but my back got so bad I was having spasms all the time. I was bent over on my right side because I had severe scoliosis. I had another back surgery in Sept of 2014. My whole back is now fused together with screws and rods. I decided to retire, except for a few clients I see out of my house. Well, within two years of being home I was back up to 197 pounds (89 kg) and had a doctor's appointment in December 2016. My doctor told me I was pre-diabetic, which didn't surprise me. My dad's side of the family all had diabetes or died from complications from diabetes. My mother had hypoglycemia most of her life. I had been tested for diabetes since I was in grade school.

I told my doctor I just didn't have any more willpower, so she told me about the ketogenic diet. In the last month of 2016, I read everything I could get my hands about this way of eating.

I was ready to start on Jan 3, 2017. It wasn't easy the first month but I never (even to this day) have eaten anything that wasn't on the plan. I keep things simple. I lost 14 pounds (6 kg) the first month, and then I stopped losing for 2 months. I didn't get discouraged because I had abused my body for so many years that I figured I was adjusting to this way of eating. I went back to the Doctor six months after I started, and she was so happy with me. My blood sugar was down to 75 mg/dl (4.2 mmol/L) and I had lost around 40 pounds (18 kg). I got off my 62 pounds (28 kg) and am down to my goal weight of 135 pounds (61 kg). I have found a new way to love and honor my body through the ketogenic diet and will eat this way for the rest of my life."[27]

Abigail wrote, "I received these before and after pictures from a friend last night as she could hardly believe the changes I have made in exactly one year. I started my journey in February 2017 and didn't take any "before" pictures because I couldn't stand to see myself in the mirror, but also because I didn't believe that I would stick with anything long enough to take a meaningful "after" photo.

I had no motivation, no dedication, and was getting very close to settling for being overweight and unhappy.

I turned 39 in February 2017 and was the heaviest I had ever been. I was so depressed, tired, suffered from panic anxiety attacks, and I was living my life on autopilot just going through the motions. I had to buy bigger clothes and when I wasn't working I was sleeping my life away. I had no motivation, no dedication, and was getting very close to settling for being overweight and unhappy. I had chronic hip and lower back pain that lead me to the chiropractor's office at least once per month. I was having terrible menstrual cycles that caused me to be extremely anemic and had to start taking a mega dose of iron every day.

Something about knocking on 40's door ignited a tiny spark in me, though. For my 39th birthday, I joined the gym that my best friend had bought the month before and I started a blind fitness quest. I had no plan, no goal, but I thought if I started working out to the point of pain every day that I would magically become a healthier person. I was so wrong. I decided I was going to be a runner and alternate cardio with heavy lifting. One month after being dedicated to the gym every day, I had shin splints that were so severe that the pain made me physically ill. I had such extreme pain in my left shoulder from improper lifting form and lifting too heavy that I could barely sleep. All of this hard work, no changes in my diet and I hadn't lost one pound in a month. I was so discouraged. I went from running on the treadmill to using the elliptical and started working out with my best friend who is also a trainer. Changing up my cardio and learning proper weightlifting techniques definitely helped, and I lost about five pounds (2.5 kg).

I went off of sugar, cold turkey the day I started the keto lifestyle.

Fast forward to October 2017. My best friend had been living in ketosis for two years and gave me some information to look into after I had voiced frustration with my inability to lose weight. Sunday, October 8th, 2017 was the first day of my two-week trial run with the ketogenic diet meal plan. This is when the game changed completely, and I started getting my life back. I had lost seven pounds (3 kg) at the end of the first week and six pounds (2.5 kg) at the end of week two. I was totally motivated and excited for more! I loved the meals that I was making and I didn't miss the sugar! I went off of sugar cold turkey the day I started the keto lifestyle.

There was only one problem: I had no endurance for cardio and couldn't do more than ten minutes on the elliptical. I couldn't lift heavy and felt like I had lost all of my strength. I just could not lift weights the first three weeks on keto. I couldn't understand what was happening! I was sleeping better at night, I had a much clearer head and was much more efficient at work, but I could not keep up in the gym. I read up on keto flu and the changes you might feel during the time of transitioning carb fuel to fat fuel and vowed to stick with it, making sure I was drinking LOTS of water and getting plenty of earthy mineral salt. I abandoned my cardio and weights routine and started taking a yoga class twice a week and completely fell in love with yoga. Amazingly, I kept losing a couple of pounds a week WITHOUT all that gym time! In November 2017 I added back a bit of cardio and weights and lo and behold my stamina was back! Not only was it back, but it was even more than before. I had made it over that hump and I felt incredible.

I feel better than I have EVER felt in my life

With the help of my friend and her gym I began my yoga instructor certification in December 2017 and was certified to teach in March 2018. Now, yoga is the only workout I do regularly besides walking my dogs daily. I haven't lifted weights, nor done that excruciating 30-45 minutes of the elliptical since December. I have lost a total of THIRTY POUNDS (14 kg) since October 8th, 2017. I weigh what I weighed at 19 years old and I turned 40 four months ago. The weight loss isn't my greatest accomplishment with keto though. My trophies are that I haven't had to see the chiropractor since October 2017. I have ZERO hip or lower-back pain! I am no longer anemic and don't take those nasty iron tabs anymore. I haven't had a single panic attack and other than that occasional rough day we all have sometimes, I have no feelings of depression! I don't nap anymore because I just don't need the sleep that I used to need. I feel better than I have EVER felt in my life. Every single day feels hopeful and full of promise. Thanks so much, keto diet."[28]

Carmella wrote, "What an amazing year it has been for me. My infant granddaughter (an identical twin) came through open heart surgery like a trooper. It was a miracle for us!

Then there was the revelation that I needed to do something about my weight. While I did not have any medical conditions diagnosed, I was just not feeling my best. These thoughts were in my mind daily... today was the day I would be good and not eat anything that might add on the pounds. The day would go on, and I would inevitably lose my willpower and eat everything in sight... Ughhhh.

I had been on several diet programs all through my 57 years, and while I may have lost some weight, it was always a struggle... and I always called it a 'diet.' I just could not keep it off. A colleague mentioned that Dr. Douglas Bishop & Associates in my city, Ottawa, Canada, had helped her lose weight and thought I should go and see them. At the beginning of February 2017, I booked my first appointment to meet Dr. Bishop, and, after a body scan and assessment by Dr. Bishop, he suggested that we try LCHF. He told me that many of his patients were doing very well with this program.

I remember sitting down with Maureen, a nurse, and my weight management counsellor, to go over the program. Well, she made it seem that I could do this, so, I would try! There were fantastic videos that helped me master the stages of LCHF and keto.

The first couple of weeks my stomach didn't like it very much, but I pushed through it. I had no idea the amount of sugar and sugar-related foods that I had previously been eating. By the time my body converted to fat burning, I was on a roll, and losing rolls at that!

There were very few weeks where I did not lose, but I persevered and the fat kept coming off. I took clothes out of my closet daily that no longer fit. I would definitely need a new wardrobe...Yes!!!

I have never mentioned willpower since because I don't think about food the same way now. I have moved more into keto as the year has progressed and really follow that old saying... I eat to live, not live to eat. I watched some videos about intermittent fasting and now fast on a regular basis, even testing 24-hour fasts at least once per week. I could never have considered fasting before, but now it seems to go hand in hand with how I am eating and living. I found yoga to be a fantastic way to reshape my body as I continue to lose fat.

My journey in the last year has seen me lose 50 pounds (23 kg), and I am close to my desired goal weight, but more than that, what I always saw myself to be. I have more energy, feel better about how I look in my clothes, and, to sum it up, I feel fantastic. My husband Greg has been so supportive and does eat LCHF most of the time. My colleagues at work and friends and family are always asking me questions about how I have done it. It's simple, go to the Diet Doctor.com site and you too can see how it can be done, and find a doctor in your area that also supports the LCHF and keto lifestyle. Having this support makes it possible to be successful. In my office alone, I have 7 colleagues that are currently doing a variety of LCHF/keto eating plans. We share recipes and ideas as to how we can convert regular foods to keto.

How I eat

I am 57 years old Bank Manager and live in Ottawa, Canada. I do intermittently fast most days and eat between noon and 8pm. About once a week, I will do a 24-hour fast and will have black coffee, broth, and water to sustain me throughout the day. This is becoming easier as I do it more often, especially if I am busy at work. The time passes and I don't even realize I have not eaten.

A couple of times a week I will eat breakfast and that would be a typical bacon and egg breakfast. Lunch is often a chicken Caesar salad that we had for dinner the previous night. As I love to go to yoga after working at the bank all day and having my meat and veggies ready to cook, makes it so much easier to ensure I stay on track. Also, I try to ensure that I have some cold cuts like roast beef, pre-cooked chicken or olives, and cheese, to make a quick dinner if I don't have time to cook.

If I go out for dinner I will often order a deconstructed burger with bacon and cheese, no bun and a side salad or a chicken Caesar salad without croutons. I don't regularly bake 'keto' desserts, but if I feel I need a little something I will have a little cream cheese with a few berries and whipped cream. It feels like I am having cheesecake without the guilt!

I find sticking with the basics, i.e. real food is so easy for me."[29]

The above testimonies have proved the effectiveness of the ketogenic diet. Although the ketogenic diet was originally developed to treat epilepsy, over the years, it has proven its versatility and its ability to evolve and treat other disorders and health issues most especially in the aspect of weight loss and keeping the body healthy and fit both mentally and physically.

Chapter Four: Why The Ketogenic Diet Works

Many people have emphasized the efficacy of the ketogenic diet and how it works wonders, but the main question that lies within is that how and why does the ketogenic diet work?

I would explain the secret behind the ketogenic diet. As it has been mentioned earlier in the previous sections, the ketogenic diet works through the process of being in a state called ketosis.

How can this state be reached? To reach the state of ketosis means that there is an absence of blood sugar in the body, which is glucose. But how can there be an absence of blood sugar since it is regarded as the fuel of the body? Can the body live without the presence of glucose? Yes, and yes, the body does well without the presence of glucose. Glucose is obtained after breaking down carbohydrate intake in the body.

This carbohydrate intake is stored in the body. Because the body can definitely not use all the intake You might be wondering and might be asking yourself, how did I gain weight? I did not consume junk like chocolates, sweets, ice cream, yet I am gaining weight? I have an answer to your questions.

You might be wondering after all has been emphasized on the effectiveness of the ketogenic diet, how does it really work and how can I be sure that it will solve my problems?

The ketogenic diet is a meal plan that consists of very low carbohydrate, minimal protein and very high in fats.

After the engagement of this diet, the body would be short on glucose, otherwise known as blood sugar, which is taken from carbohydrates. At this moment, there is nothing to "*fuel*" the body. The fat you consume, and the fat you stored previously, when broken down, will produce fatty acids and ketones.

These ketones would be transferred around the body and then transported to the brain. It assumes the work of glucose without issues. When it reaches a certain point in this engagement, the body's fuel supply is solely on ketones. This state is known as ketosis.

Ketosis is known for its efficacy in weight reduction and solving other disorders. During its inception, the ketogenic diet was and is still known for its effectiveness in treating epilepsy.

At this moment, there is nothing to *"fuel"* the body. The fat you consume, and the fat you stored previously, when broken down, will produce fatty acids and ketones.

These ketones would be transferred around the body and then transported to the brain. It assumes the work of glucose without issues. When it reaches a certain point in this engagement, the body's fuel supply is solely on ketones. This state is known as ketosis.

Ketosis is known for its efficacy in weight reduction and solving other disorders. During its inception, the ketogenic diet was and is still known for its effectiveness in treating epilepsy.

Misconceptions And Wrong Thoughts About Ketogenic Diet

The ketogenic is widely accepted by all and this is due to its effectiveness. This has made a lot of people question its goodness and therefore developed a lot of misconceptions from it.

Some of these misconceptions are from people's ignorance, their fears and also the fact that keto can do the seemingly impossible, which makes it so hard for them to believe. Below are but a few misconceptions people have in regards to the ketogenic diet:

YOU CAN CONSUME AS MUCH FAT AS YOU WANT

Being on a keto diet does not give you the free rein to eat as much fat as you wish just to get your fats in. Although about 75% of your meal in a keto diet should be fat, that does not mean you can eat as many saturated fats as you so desire.

Unsaturated fats are actually the preferred and recommended option by dieticians and health professionals; it has also been confirmed by studies and research. IT IS REALLY DANGEROUS

There have been a lot of speculations that the ketogenic diet is very dangerous. This can happen to people who do not follow the ketogenic diet judiciously and to heart.

It has been said to cause a mineral deficiency, a high increase in cholesterol level and so on. It has also been said to cause heart disease. All these can be duly avoided if you hit and know your macros and micronutrients daily and you also ensure that you stay hydrated, and then all these downsides can be totally avoided and disarmed.

KETOSIS AND KETOACIDOSIS ARE TOTALLY THE SAME

The belief that ketosis and ketoacidosis are the same has been roaming all around but the two are totally different. "Ketosis is the metabolic process of using fat as the primary source of energy instead of carbohydrates. This means your body is directly breaking down its fat stores as energy instead of slowly converting fat and muscle cells into glucose for energy."[30]

That was according to Perfect Keto. Ketoacidosis, on the other hand, can be seen in diabetic patients who follow the ketogenic diet. Ketoacidosis is a "condition resulting from dangerously high levels of ketones and blood sugar," according to Healthline. This causes the blood to become too acidic, and it affects organ function.

KETOGENIC DIET IS A HIGH PROTEIN DIET

The ketogenic diet is not a high protein diet. A ketogenic diet should consist of 75% fat, 20% protein, and 5% carbohydrate. If it were to be a high protein diet, it would have a protein percentage of between 30-35%.

FASTING IS A REQUIREMENT FOR KETO DIET

This is one I would like to really lay emphasis on. Fasting is not a requirement for ketogenic diet. It is not recommended to add fasting to your diet until you are already used to the system.

However, intermittent fasting alongside the ketogenic diet has its own benefits. It increases detoxification, weight loss and it also helps you reduce cravings and hunger. It should be well noted that you do not engage in intermittent fasting alongside your keto diet unless you have mastered the diet like reducing your carbohydrate intake level.

KETO DIET IS ALCOHOL RESISTANCE

Being in the ketogenic diet does not really mean alcohol should be totally avoided. Although most wines and alcohols are high carbohydrate sources, some alcohols are very low in carbohydrates, keto friendly like gin, vodka etc.

Alcohol should not be totally removed from the question but all is required of you is to be conscious of what you choose and be careful of how you drink while on the keto diet. It is important for you to note that your alcohol tolerability would be lower while you are on a ketogenic diet.

KETOGENIC DIET IS ONLY GOOD FOR WEIGHT LOSS

This is one of the persistent ketogenic diet myths and misconception. This belief connotes that the ketogenic diet is only and solely beneficial for people who are engaging in it for the purpose of weight loss. Do not be confused here, I did not say ketogenic diet is not useful for weight loss; it is a great and very effective tool for weight reduction but it can do a lot more.

Studies haves shown that the ketogenic diet promotes weight loss and it also helps to counteract many vices that increase risk of heart disease and some metabolic symptoms. Not only this, but it has also proven to:

- Likely increase the lifespan
- To decrease food and sugar cravings
- To increase energy levels
- To increase mitochondrial health
- To ease inflammatory skin conditions
- Reduce the probability of having several chronic diseases like diabetes, chronic fatigue, cancer, neurodegeneration
- Cuts system inflammation

THE BRAIN NEEDS SUGAR TO FUNCTION

This misconception is really common amidst a great percentage of the world's population. The belief that the brain needs sugar to function and be able to perform effectively.

Thus, glucose is referred to as the fuel of the body. The illogical reasoning behind this is that glucose is taken from the carbohydrates we take in and the ketogenic diet promotes a drastic reduction in the intake of carbohydrates, so if the intake of carbohydrate which is the source of glucose reduces greatly, the body and brain will not function properly and effectively.

The ignorance in this is that the increase and decrease in fats and carbohydrates respectively are very beneficial to the body, and the fats, when broken down, produces ketone bodies which effectively replaces the glucose in the fuelling and effective functionality of the brain.

It carries out the work of the subsidized glucose and brings along added advantages like improvement in mental alertness, cognition. It has been shown by studies that the ketogenic diet has huge benefits in reducing the symptoms in Alzheimer's patients, and this is achieved by switching the brain to work on ketones instead of glucose.

Above are various examples of misconceptions regarding the ketogenic diet. The above have are facts against those misconceptions.

If you have any other questions regarding the ketogenic diet or you have concepts that seem misty or unclear, you should visit a dietician or a health professional.

This brings us to the end of the chapter, in light of the above segments; the meaning of ketogenic diet has been duly explained.

The history and development of the ketogenic diet have been explained as well.

You have learned that the ketogenic diet was originally invented for the treatment of epilepsy and seizures in little children but along the way, it was discovered that it does a lot more than the treatment of epilepsy.

The process behind the ketogenic diet has also been explained. How it works, what is required for this to happen? We have also laid emphasis on the various misconceptions of people regarding the ketogenic diet like the belief that you can eat as much fat as you want, and the misconception that the ketogenic diet is very dangerous. All these have been rebutted and well explained.

Chapter Five: Why You Should Engage In Ketogenic Diet And Intermittent Fasting For Weight Loss

I have received a lot of questions regarding the use of the ketogenic diet. Many people ask, why should I engage in this ketogenic diet? How is it better than other weight loss programs? Why should I fast to lose weight? Is it logical to do so? How does it work? Is it really effective?

Tom is a 61-year-old man who weighs 87 kg. When he was 59 years old, he was an obese man with high blood pressure, high cholesterol and so on. His doctors were thrilled that he reduced weight drastically and not only that, there was a significant change in his life.

People were wondering what gave him such drive, was it because a friend of his died recently? Or was it because there was a reunion coming up? All these were true but are not the reason.

Tom has a daughter named Alina; she is 28 years old. She was working successfully as an accountant. She was happy and successful. Alina had occasional headaches but the doctors did not pay attention to it. In September 2016, she was rushed to the emergency room. The doctors found a massive tumor in her brain. She had two surgeries to remove the tumor. The news was that she was suffering from glioblastoma. It is an aggressive fast-growing brain cancer. The average survival for this was 12 months.

After the surgery, they decided to join a ketogenic diet study. It is not expected, right? Who prescribes that for a cancer treatment?

But this was not a random decision made; they found out through research that the ketogenic diet treats cancer. Now they could have gone through any other therapy and treatments. Tom, who was obese, could have done several other things but why ketogenic diet? Tom joined Alina as her coach and chef.

The ketogenic diet does not entirely cure cancer but the diet has shown promise for some cancers especially GBM. How is this so? On a simplistic level, cancer eats glucose and needs 20 times more glucose compared to other cells. Cancer cells cannot make the transition to using ketones, especially in the brain, making them more vulnerable to chemo and radiation.

The first two weeks for them was hard to start with. They gave up a lot of comfort foods. So, switching to a ketogenic diet is not the first thing that pops to your head when you hear cancer but the diet works. Tom steadily lost weight without substantial hunger or changes to his exercise program. His overall health improved drastically, he slept better and the change I mentioned earlier was that his daughter Alina, today, is a cancer survivor.

They are now two years behind her initial diagnosis and there has been no evidence of tumor regrowth. The ketogenic diet has really helped them overcome their challenges. Tom has lost 48 kg.

The evident reasoning here is that they could have done other therapies but the ketogenic diet came to their rescue.

The ketogenic diet and intermittent fasting are always easier means of weight reduction. I could remember the case of an obese boy who was bullied and mocked in school.

At all cost, he wanted to lose weight but whenever he went jogging, people would always make fun of him; if he went to the gym in his school, his mates bullied and it was kind of embarrassing for him because he was socially mocked and this affected him psychologically.

He was not mentally inclined any longer. He was introduced to the ketogenic diet and intermittent fasting; such a relief!

He was no longer laughed at while reducing weight because all he did was private. Nobody knew what he was eating, the number of carbohydrates he took in. And with time, he lost 30kg. He was no longer bullied and ridiculed.

If your story or situation is similar to the boy, it is never too late to begin. If you have been shamed and mocked for your situation, the ketogenic diet is here for you. It is not compulsory that people know you are going through a weight reduction scheme. You can also engage in intermittent fasting in the confines of your room and nobody would know about it.

Most people lose on their weight loss schemes due to many reasons. A friend of mine misses her gym class due to prolonged meetings until I made her know the efficacy of ketogenic diet and intermittent fasting. She does not have to leave meetings. Many of you are trying to lose weight but because of your busy schedule and work, you cannot easily accomplish your fitness goals. Why bother? The ketogenic diet is here for you.

Some of you have very busy and time-consuming professions, like bankers, accountants, engineers, doctors and so on. For example, a banker who has to be in front of a desk all day attending to customers has no time to schedule for his or her fitness and weight reduction schemes.

Why not go through the ketogenic diet and also fast intermittently? This will not hinder your job effectiveness or time schedule, but would rather boost your mental alertness, your cognitive development and would really increase your work efficiency.

Is that not a great and effortless offer? All you have to do is to take the step and discover a world of ease and great outcome.

Other Weight Loss Programs That You Can Replace With The Ketogenic Diet And Intermittent Fasting

There are weight loss programs that the ketogenic diet and intermittent fasting can substitute. This may be due to various reasons and influencing factors. Let us examine some of these below and try to understand why this is so.

Going to the gym

It is evident that whenever someone says that he or she wants to lose some weight, the first statement that family and friends would say is, *"why not hit the gym?"*

This is why you can get your desired body and you can work out your fitness goals. I would be laying down some sample cases and we would have to decide at the end of the day.

A woman that is unemployed goes to the gym to work out daily and reach her fitness goals. Fortunately for her, she got a job into a firm a company as their lawyer. So the woman will not be able to go to the gym again.

You might be wondering why this is so? She would have several cases and preparations, she would be so busy that there will not be time for her to hit the gym, and over time she gains weight.

Although she is making money, and this is good, there is a saying I love that says *"health is wealth."*

She is not able to take care of her health again. Sometimes if she comes back from work late at night, she would be so tired to cook and she would eat junk.

All this can be solved through the introduction of the ketogenic diet. She would not have to make time out of her busy schedule and eat junk again but still, she is losing weight.

Our second case is that of a movie producer. It is evident that movie producers have to spend most of their time on set and locations.

Such an individual will not be able to go to the gym and therefore his or her fitness goals are gradually ruined. Why not go into intermittent fasting: most directors don't have a problem with missing or skipping meals. There are various times they would have to shoot some scenes by 3am. They can continually shoot a scene throughout the morning and even forget they have not eaten. Is that not an opportunity? That is a means of turning a demerit into an added advantage. All you have to do is to draw out a plan but it is advisable to see a doctor before you commence in order to know if you can do it or not. The ketogenic diet has made weight loss very easy.

Use of herbal medicines and drugs

You might be wondering how the ketogenic diet and intermittent fasting would supplement or replace this. It would be such a great feeling of joy and happiness if you realize that a single drug can make you lose and shed weight.

The stress of going to the gym and so on would be uplifted. Even in our society today, such drugs are rampant. The government will do anything in its capacity to subsidize the price of such drugs because the result it brings is very enticing. It reduces the rate at which people develop heart diseases and this indirectly reduces the rate at which people die in society. But with that, some of them are still quite exorbitant in price. We are going to look at the case of a woman named Grace.

Grace is an accountant. She is very successful and quite diligent at everything she does. She is very resourceful. Grace went to learn culinary arts and cooking. She was the catch to all men's eyes.

But unfortunately for those men, she was in a relationship. But then her boyfriend broke up with her which really left Grace devastated. It was a relationship of 5 years. She cried for weeks. She had only one companion that kept her through those times: it was junk food.

After she got over the trauma of the heartbreak, she could not get over the way she now eats junk. She ate junk and could not stop it.

With time, she started gaining a lot of weight, her waistline increased massively. The once beautiful Grace, the aim of all men became just *"adorable"*. This was brought to her friends' notice and they told her about a herbal drug that reduces the weight of its users.

She was very happy that she found a solution to her problems at last. What a relief! She started taking the herbal pill but still, there was no improvement. Instead she still gained more and more weight. You might be wondering why this is so? The problem she has is not with her body but with her habit. The drug she was using was to make her a change in her body but the causative factors was still left untreated.

She was later introduced to the ketogenic diet and intermittent fasting. This totally worked because the problem she was having was not with her body but with her habit, and the ketogenic diet changes your habit and lifestyle because it is not just a diet, it is a lifestyle.

This also relates to most people who are solely dependent on drugs and see no improvement. The problem is not your body system, but your habitual trait which can only be corrected by a remedy that deals with a lifestyle approach and this is the ketogenic diet.

So what are you waiting for? It is never too late to start. I believe in the saying that goes thus, *"A journey of a thousand miles begins with a step."*

Jogging and other forms of exercise

This system of body fitness and weight reduction is mostly used by everybody but is it really everybody? Waking up in the morning, if you look outside your window, you would see a lot of people, most especially your neighbors, going for a jog.

You wish you could join them as before but why is this not so. We might have the same traits as human beings but we are quite peculiar in our different ways. As our fingerprints do not match with any other person's own, so are our traits.

You wish you could also lace up your shoes every morning and go out for a jog. Not everybody is inclined to that. Some of us cannot afford to go for a mile jog and still have to get to the office very early in the morning. We are going to look at three sample cases in our plot.

Abigail is a very athletic person in school. She has got the shape and the brains. She ran track in high school and is a very good jogger. She is always after her body fitness and how to stay healthy. Now she is married with two kids. After she had her first child, she resorted to going back into jogging and keeping fit until she realized she was already pregnant again.

She did not have time for herself again, she had to take care of the children, prepare breakfast early in the morning, and she lost the zeal for early morning jogging. She started gaining some extra weight because she was stress eating.

The problem she has now is that she has a college reunion coming up in 5 months and it would be so embarrassing if her mates see that the once ever fit Abigail is now an obese woman. What can she do?

Abraham is a banker. He is very fit and also a body trainer. On one of his meetings with a client, he had an accident. This was a very terrible accident. He almost lost his legs. He was no longer on wheelchairs but he cannot walk for a long time. This made him really down; he ate and consumed junk in all kinds and forms. He is becoming quite obese and his fiancée is about to break up with him unless he loses some weight. What can he do?

Richard is very reactive to how he looks and what he puts into his body; his friends call him a fitness freak. Richard lost it all when he lost his parents and siblings in a car crash. He was the only one that survived the crash. He lost one of his legs and he became frustrated. It was so bad that he tried committing suicide. He ate and ate. Now he has found redemption and love through a woman he refers to as his God-sent angel. He is now overweight. He wants to make a difference in his weight, but how can he do it?

To Abigail, I know being a mother is quite tiring and time-consuming but you have got to do all it takes. It is not really compulsory for you to jog before you can lose but have you not heard of the ketogenic diet? You do not have to jog again, just form a meal plan for your diet and start following it judiciously and I can assure you that before your college reunion you would be even fit than you used to be. So start the ketogenic diet today and you would see the difference.

To Abraham, I would advise you to not stress yourself too much since you are still recuperating. You need to see a doctor in order to know if you are fit to start the ketogenic diet because of your status. If you are approved to do so, it would be a wonderful experience because you would be amazed at the outcome. I would advise you not to add intermittent fasting alongside the ketogenic diet because of situations whereby you have to use drugs and supplements.

To Richard, I know you were hurting and you did not have control over your habits. I know for sure that you still have a purpose and it must be fulfilled. It is quite nice, the way you want to redeem yourself. It is a very simple thing because I have a remedy for you. The ketogenic diet is very effective in such cases. You have to be diligent and follow it strictly and I am sure you would have yourself redeemed and you will have no reason to feel depressed about life and its challenges.

It has been shown in our cases above that the ketogenic diet is very effective in replacing jogging for people with some peculiarities.

Employing the use of work-out videos

Not everybody is able to go to a gym and workout or meet their fitness goals. This may be due to various reasons. To some, it is the stress of having to go to the gym. And to some other people, it is the unavailability of time. To most other people, it is due to the fact that they do not want to be mocked by others in the gym or while jogging. So they resort to the use of workout DVD. Most people cannot afford to pay the fee to gym classes, so why not use an affordable DVD instead?

The workout DVD is very affordable and you can do it in the confines of your home. But is there a disadvantage to this? We are going to look at the stories of two or three people in order for us to understand better.

Leslie is a sales representative of a pharmaceutical company. She is uptight and all about her weight. She could not afford the fee to be a member of the gym so she bought a workout DVD and she started her fitness journey.

Very good news hit her and she was very delighted about this. She was being considered for a promotion at work. She began to work over her schedule in order to impress the management and be given the promotion. She gradually stopped having time for herself and her body. She added some pounds to her weight due to the fact that she did not have time to cook again, all she ate was junk. At times during the weekend, when she's tired, she treats herself to a late night snack of chicken and a bag of potato chips. She gained 15 pounds. When she realized the changes in her weight, she was petrified that she was going to lose the promotion. What is she to do?

Danny is a lawyer. He has three kids and a beautiful wife. Few years into their marriage, he gained some weight and this was due to the stress of having to provide for the family and fend for the extended family. Due to his busy schedule, he could not apply to a gym but his wife bought him a workout DVD to use. This was great news to him. He started using the workout DVD and it was effective. He was then offered to be a partner, but it was still months away. He started doing everything in his power to make sure he got the partnership because he had competitors. He had totally forgotten about the workout DVD and started gaining more weight. This was to his surprise; he did not want his wife to come back and meet him obese, because she traveled. He was left in a confusing state, the reason being that if his wife came back and met him obese she would not take it lightly with him and if he starts working out, he will not have time to chase his lifetime opportunity of being a partner. What will he do?

Hillary is a very successful woman. She has three kids and a loving husband. Unfortunately, her husband died in an accident. She was left all alone with three kids; she was very depressed and stressed out. She had to take care of the children and also fend for herself. She gained a lot of weight. On realizing this, she went to register at a gym but on hearing the time schedule, she could not make it. So, she bought a workout DVD and started the fitness program but along the line, she could not carry on due to the responsibilities on her alone. She gained more and more weight. She is wondering about the way out for her. What will she do?

To all three sides, this is a very compromising condition. For the case of Leslie, as I have said earlier, health is wealth. Do not deprive yourself of good health all because you want wealth.

I have a solution to your worries. You do not have to worry or give yourself unnecessary stress because the ketogenic diet is here to help. The problem is the unavailability of time, so you need a measure that does not take valuable time away from you. You can be on the ketogenic diet and still have enough time for your promotion goals to work out. All you have to do is to control your carbohydrate intake, minimize the amount of protein you take in and increase your fat intake. I can assure you of a positive outcome and a well-fitted body to take up that promotion.

To Danny, life is full of various solutions; you just have to explore it. I would proffer a solution that is well tested and trusted to you. The ketogenic diet, started today, and your wife would meet a completely different man compared to what she left and you would be surprised yourself.

To Hillary, I know life might be hard sometimes but do not let it bring you down or diminish who you are. Try the ketogenic diet today and you would see the difference.

I know that these cases might relate to you in one way or the other. The ketogenic diet is here for you. Not alone will it fight your weight problems but also treat other disorders in your body.

Chapter Six: Benefits Of Intermittent Fasting

In the world of health and health management, intermittent fasting is coming back to fame and popular recognition. The history of intermittent fasting could be traced back to the dawn of man. It has been a great advantage to man. Below are some of the benefits of intermittent fasting:

1. It improves fat burning
2. It increases weight and body fat loss
3. It increases your energy level
4. It lowers sugar levels and blood insulin
5. It improves mental clarity and concentration
6. It reverses type 2 diabetes
7. It increases the growth hormone
8. It lowers the blood cholesterol level
9. It potentially elongates the lifespan
10. It reduces inflammation.

1. IMPROVES FAT BURNING

This is one of the main benefits of intermittent fasting. It rapidly increases the rate at which fats in the body burns. The schedule of your fasting burns fats. The fats in your body are caused by excess carbohydrates that are stored up. So, not eating at intervals will reduce the rate at which you eat, and this will reduce your fat level.

2. IT INCREASES WEIGHT AND BODY FAT LOSS

The intermittent fasting weight loss programs have been known for effectiveness in the rapid loss of weight by its users, and it also reduces body fat. It is trending now because of its outcome and various testimonies people have made. It reduces the rate at which you eat, therefore reducing your body weight and fat.

3. IT INCREASES YOUR ENERGY LEVEL

You might be wondering how fasting which is quite tiring to you makes you get energy. The main reason for being overweight is because of the unused carbohydrate that has been stored up. So being on an intermittent fasting schedule would definitely reduce the fat and the rest would be fully which will promote a faster generation of energy. Furthermore, if the body is enlightened from the excess fat in it, it will be able to carry out more functions. Also, as the saying goes, *"A healthy body is an agile body."*

4. IT LOWERS SUGAR LEVELS AND BLOOD INSULIN

Studies have shown that intermittent fasting reduces the level of blood sugar in the body. Intermittent fasting as a process in which the level of eating is limited during certain times of the week helps men and women to lose a massive amount of weight and also helps in reducing their insulin. Oftentimes, diabetes is treated as a drug-related condition not with therapies and diet, and treating it with drugs never addresses the root of the problem of diabetes. Weight has been said to help people reduce insulin resistance and it also helps to absorb blood sugar more effectively.

5. IT IMPROVES MENTAL CLARITY AND CONCENTRATION

This is a crucial benefit that intermittent fasting brings to man. The shedding of excess weight and fat makes the cognitive development increase rapidly. Let us look at a story of Tony. Tony is a high school kid but he is obese and he was always mocked and bullied by his mates. He was introduced to intermittent fasting by one of his mother's friends. After weeks of the therapy, his life changed. His self-confidence increased and his attention to his studies also. His fears were alleviated and he began to excel in class. He was mentally alert.

It has been proven that intermittent fasting increases the rate at which we think. Some experts have explained that most obese patients have issues with depression and tend to always feel down about themselves, but on losing weight, those fears and depression will be uplifted and this brings about more alertness mentally.

In most cases, this is mostly not true, the reason being that the reduction in the way we eat also helps our brain increase its functionality and thereby promoting alertness and sharpness in the person.

6. IT REVERSES TYPE TWO DIABETES

It is a great advantage to the world that intermittent fasting reverses this condition. Type 2 diabetes is caused by the body's resistance to insulin and increased blood sugar.

These are some of the benefits derived while doing intermittent fasting. It reduces the blood cholesterol level. It also elongates the lifespan through the treatment of blood sugar level, blood cholesterol level, and it has also been known to treat Alzheimer's disease and other syndromes.

The benefits of intermittent fasting take a long and large catalog and cannot be mentioned in words but rather through experience. So, why not start today and see its various benefits.

Benefits Of The Ketogenic Diet

The benefits of the ketogenic diet have a large catalog. The ketogenic diet provides a long range of benefits and treatments. When it was invented, the sole purpose was to cure and treat seizures in little children.

The ketogenic diet came into limelight when testimony was shared by Charlie Abrahams. Research and studies have shown that the ketogenic diet rapidly reduces the weight of the patient.

Below are but a few benefits of the ketogenic diet:

1] The ketogenic diet has its efficacy in the reduction of weight and body fat. The reduction of weight and body fat in the body while engaging in the ketogenic diet is through the state of ketosis. Ketosis has been known to drastically reduce body weight because, during this state, the body fats that have been stored up will be burned up and be used, thereby causing a large reduction of weight in the body of such individual. To get into this state of ketosis is not quite easy but it can be achieved through the ketogenic diet. The ketogenic diet increases fat intake, and when they are broken down, will bring out ketones that serve this purpose.

2] The ketogenic diet increases the mental agility and alertness of its patients. This has been proved by various people that have benefitted from the ketogenic diet. As explained in the previous chapter, the ketogenic diet reduces depression in its patients which makes them more active. By the mere absence of the blood sugar, the ketogenic diet helps the functionality of the brain which makes the brain function better and increases the cognitive prowess of such an individual.

3] The ketogenic aids the control of the blood sugar level. The ketogenic diet aids the reduction and the perfect control of blood sugar level. The meal structure of the ketogenic diet tells it all. The sugar in the blood is caused by the excess intake of carbohydrates and the ketogenic diet curbs this by making a meal plan that reduces the intake of carbohydrates we take in and increases the number of fats.

4] The ketogenic diet has mastery in the treatment of seizures in epileptic patients, especially small children. Tracing the history of the ketogenic diet, it can be found that the ketogenic diet was originally designed to treat seizures and reduce the chances in little children. This has been a great help to the human race at the same time. Even when the anticonvulsant drugs fail, medical practitioners resort to the ketogenic diet for help.

5] The ketogenic diet also treats disorders and diseases like the Alzheimer's disease, heart disease, fatty liver, and numerous diseases.

6] The ketogenic diet has been proven to elongate and increase one's lifespan. This might be surprising to you but studies have shown that this is certified and authentic. The alleviation and reduction in weight and body fat reduce the rate at which one becomes a victim of life-taking diseases. The ketogenic diet through its effective treatment of seizures in epileptic patients and this has been known to reduce the rate at which the disease becomes deadly.

In light of the above, the benefits that the ketogenic diet brings to its patients are quite convincing that it is the perfect diet for you. So, why not try it out today and you would see that your life will never remain the same!

Chapter Seven: Different Types And Kinds Of Intermittent Fasting

The intermittent fasting varies in types and has many diverse ways of doing and engaging in it. Below are some different ways to go about intermittent fasting:

1] The 16/8 method: This is fasting for 16 hours each day. This method as I have said earlier involves the fasting for 14-16 hours and solely restricts your eating window to 8-10 hours each day.

With this, one is permitted to eat around 2-3 meals. This method of fasting is also known as the Leangains protocol and this was propounded and popularized by fitness expert Martin Berkhan. This method is as easy as not eating anything for dinner or skipping breakfast.

For example, if you eat dinner around 8 pm, all you have to do is to not eat anything until 12 noon the following the day. This makes you technically fasted for 16 hours. It is advised that women should only fast 14-15 hours because they do much better with slightly shorter fasts.

This might be really hard and not easy to adhere to by people who are fond of eating in the morning or having late night snacks. It will be very comfortable for people who skip breakfast because that is essentially how they eat.

If you are not quite comfortable with the early morning hunger, you can take water, coffee, and other beverages. They also serve as a means of reducing hunger levels and the temptation of sneaking in a snack for you.

You should note that it is of utmost importance to eat very healthy foods during your window period. The fact that you are engaging in intermittent fasting does not warrant you to eat excess junk. Consuming a lot of calories during your window period is likely to hinder the effects of the intermittent fasting.

Personally, I find this to be the most natural way of fasting because I also do it. It has been proven that late night snacks are not extensively digested by our digestive system, thereby causing a redundant amount of excess fats and calories not burned in our body.

This is also effortless; not only are you doing your digestive system a favor, but you are also benefiting from it in several other ways. Let me use myself as an example, I also engage in the ketogenic diet, so I am really not hungry until around 1 pm in the afternoon. Later on, I eat my last meal around 6-9pm. With this, I end up fasting for 16-19 hours each day.

The summary and bottom line of this is that the 16/8 method consists of daily fasting of 16 hours for men and advisably 14-15 hours for women. This leaves you with an 8-hour window of eating which will range 2-3 meals.

It is highly advisable not to take advantage of this window and eat excess junk or take in too many calories. This will hinder the effectiveness of the fasting and results may not be as you expected.

2] The 5:2 diet: this means that you will fast for 2 days a week. This involves you eating normally for 5 days and then fasting for the remaining 2 days whereby you restrict your intake of calories between the ranges of 500-600.

This is also known as the fast diet. It was popularized by a renowned doctor and a British journalist Michael Mosley. It is advisable that women eat 500 calories and men eat 600 calories on these fasting days.

For example, you might decide that the two days you want to fast are on Mondays and Wednesdays. So it is expected that on these days you eat two meals each consisting 250 calories for women and each consisting 300 calories for men. As critics rightly pointed out, there is no valid study testing this diet but there are many studies and research that have tested and proven the intermittent fasting to be effective and very useful in the reduction of weight and other benefits. So we can rightly say since this diet is a form of intermittent fasting, it can be said to be effective and reliable.

The bottom line of what is above is that the intermittent fasting involves eating 500 calories for women and 600 calories for men for two days of the week but they can freely eat normally for the other 5 days that are left.

3] Eat-Stop-Eat: It means the fasting is done for 24 hours. This approach to intermittent fasting involves the fasting for 24 hours once or twice a week. This method was popularized by the renowned fitness expert Brad Pilon and this method has been in trend for quite some years now.

If you fast from dinner today to dinner tomorrow, it means you have fasted for 24 hours. For example, if you finish eating dinner by 8 pm on Friday and you do not eat until 8 pm on Saturday, it means that you have fasted for 24 hours straight. The option used in the 16/8 diet can also be used due to the longevity in the fast. Non-caloric beverages like coffee, water and so on can be taken during the fast but no solid food is allowed during the fast. The reason is that those beverages have been known to be a very useful tool in reducing hunger level. Therefore, they reduce the rate of temptations to break the fast.

If you are doing this to lose weight, it is very important to note that, it is very crucial to eat normally during your window period. The fact that you just fasted for 24 hours does not warrant you to eat excessively on your non-fasting days. So, the amount of food should be minimized.

One of the biggest problems of this form of intermittent fasting is that it is very difficult to follow since it is for a full 24 hours. You might be wondering how you would go into it right away. It is not compulsory to start straight away, you can start with 14-16 hours and then you can move upward from there. I can testify to this, I have done it a few times.

The beginning would be very easy but the ending hours will be like hell. That is why I went to the 14-16 hours and now it has increased to 16-19 hours. So, it is not really something that you start up straight away.

In a few words, the Eat-Stop-Eat method of intermittent fasting involves a fasting routine which entails 24 hours fast for one or two days each week.

4] Alternate Day fasting: The alternate day fasting means that you fast every other day. There are many versions of this method. Most of them allow about 500 calories when you are on your fasting days. Various labs studies that show the benefits of intermittent fasting used some versions of this method. A full fast every other day seems too extreme, so I really do not recommend this for beginners.

Going through this method, you will be going to your bed hungry many times each week. This is not really pleasant and it is quite unsustainable on a long-term basis.

The Alternate day fasting simply means that you are fasting every other day, it can be by not eating anything at all or by eating a few hundred calories.

5] The Warrior diet: This name might sound absurd for a diet but it means fasting during the day and eating a huge meal at night. This diet method was popularized by a fitness expert named Ori Hofmekler. This diet involves you eating a small or minimal amount of vegetables and fruits during the day and eating one huge meal at night. This basically means that you fast all day and you feast at night within a 4-hour window.

This diet was one of the popular diets to include the intermittent fasting. This diet has also been said to embrace food choices that are closely related to the paleo diet. From my point of view, this diet has a history which has been depicted by the name. Warrior diet can be similarly traced to the ancient times when the warriors would leave for battlefield early in the morning. They would only eat a few things they can find on the way like fruits and vegetables. After the battle, they would return at night and, merry, feast like kings. They would eat a lot and sleep. The cycle begins the next day all over.

In essence, the warrior diet is all about eating little amounts of fruits and vegetables during the day and eating a huge meal in the night within a 4-hour eating window.

6] Spontaneous meal skipping: This simply means that you skip meals when it is convenient. This means that you do not have to follow a structured fasting plan, all you have to do is to skip meals when it is convenient for you. You can skip meals from time to time when you are probably too busy or you just do not feel like eating.

There is a myth that tells that humans have to eat from time to time or they will lose their muscle and reach starvation mode. As you might have well understood now, the human body is well structured and equipped to handle extended periods of famine, not to talk about missing one or two meals from time to time. It is quite easy to do, if you are not hungry, you can skip breakfast, or if you are in heavy traffic, instead of buying roadside snacks, why not do a short fast.

Not eating one or two meals is what spontaneous intermittent fasting implies. Make sure you eat healthy foods during meals.

To cap it all, spontaneous fasting is the most natural way to do intermittent fasting and this is just by skipping one or two meals when you do not feel like eating or when you do not even have time to eat.

We have been able to examine various methods and approach to intermittent fasting. The question now is, how do I know the one that I will do? Just choose the one that is most convenient for you or you can seek the help of a dietician, a health professional and so on. Choose and start one today and you would never be the same!

Different Types Of The Ketogenic Diet

The ketogenic diet varies in types; there are various approaches by which someone can do the ketogenic diet and reach a state of ketosis.

There are many types of ketogenic diets and each one of them is useful for different purposes.

You will compare each of them and then decide the path that you will take in order to reach your fitness goals. I will be sharing some of these approaches and types ketogenic diet to you. Below are the approaches and types of ketogenic diet:

1] The Standard ketogenic diet [SKD]: The standard ketogenic diet is the most basic form of the ketogenic diet. The goal of the SKD is to have 50 grams or less of carbohydrates each day in order to keep you in a state of ketosis. Your calories will be obtained from fats and proteins. This is actually the best place to get started with your diet and due to its effectiveness many people who have tested it have no reason to change to another type because of the positive results they got.

2] The Targeted ketogenic diet [TKD]: The aim of the Targeted ketogenic diet is to have you consume your carbohydrates during your workout times. It can be immediately before or immediately after your workout time.

This plan of diet is most useful to people that do workouts and exercise regularly. It can be the new athletes or it can be the ones that are highly trained. The carbohydrates should be kept very low, even though the workouts can increase carbohydrate tolerance. It is mostly done by people by consuming 30-50 grams of carbohydrate in order to maintain their energy levels during a workout.

3] The Cyclic ketogenic diet [CKD]: The cyclic ketogenic diet is mainly for advanced athletes that need a greater boost in carbohydrates for fuel during their training. These types of athletes include power lifters, endurance runners and professional players. They would consume a high level of carbohydrate for two days before their competition in order to fully reload their glycogen storage. This will really help them in their muscle growth and also their power, although it can also lead to fat storage.

4] The High protein ketogenic diet: This model of the ketogenic diet is mainly for the people that want to shed excess body fat. In the high protein ketogenic diet, the aim is to drop excess fat not just body weight from the body in general.

Through having a higher proportion of protein compared to fats, the body would be able to keep a lean muscle mass and to build muscle in the case of working out. To also make sure to use the fat that is already stored up in the body as fuel and this is even faster than the normal ketogenic diet. On this model, you would consume up to 1.5 grams of protein per pound of lean mass. This increase in protein to burn fats faster and makes it easier to lose fat while maintaining and gaining strength.

5] The Protein Sparing Modified Fast [PSMF]: This is a highly restrictive modification of the ketogenic diet. It includes mainly lean proteins and it is kept to 600-1000 calories a day. It is designed as a temporary solution to kick-start weight loss while preserving the muscle mass. Those that are on it avoid meat that is essentially higher in fat. Do not add fat while cooking and continue to avoid carbohydrates. The fat that produces the ketone bodies comes mainly from the fats that are stored up in the body. This model is a great temporarily; it is not sustainable as a lifestyle to its users.

Chapter Eight: Choosing The Perfect Intermittent Fasting For You

In light of the chapters before, you have seen various types of intermittent fasting and several approaches to them. It has been observed by psychologists that one of the uncertainties that reside in man are the inability to know the journey or challenge for him to engage in.

This is really hard, I know because there are various options to pick or select from and this is quite confusing. That is why I am here to help you go through this and achieve your prospective fitness goals.

As I have mentioned in the previous chapter, the intermittent fasting varies in methods and styles by which people approach it. I made mention of these methods, which include:

1] 16/8 method of fasting: This involves you fasting for 14-16 hours a day.

2] 5:2 diets: This involves fasting for 2 days a week.

3] Eat-Stop-Eat: This involves you fasting 24 hours for one or two days per week.

4] Alternate day fasting: This involves you fasting for every other day.

5] Warrior diet: This is an approach that can literally be likened to a warrior; it involves eating of fruits and vegetable throughout the day and eating a huge meal at night.

6] Spontaneous method: This happens to each and every one of us. It simply means skipping meals intentionally and occasionally when you are not really hungry or you are quite busy at work and other things. This is one of the most natural ways of carrying out the intermittent fasting.

There are various reasons that push people into carrying out the intermittent fasting. Some do it to shed weight, some to stay healthy; others do it to keep fit. There is a twist in this decision making, how would you know the perfect one for you? Let us look at a case.

Rebecca is a sales rep. She was quite surprised when she got on the scale and realized that she weighs 176 pounds. She was terrified and confused about how it happened. She went online and read some articles and books on losing weight. Then she saw an article about the intermittent fasting and its numerous advantages. She decided to do it. She also decides to be on the warrior diet because it looked promising and she thought it would yield a faster result that would help her to reach her fitness goals.

On the first day of her fast, the first hours were quite easy, she felt happy. But due to the nature of her job, she needed the energy to keep on. She started fading out and losing balance by 3 pm. Oh no, she must get something to eat. She rushed down to the nearest place she could get food and she ate. So sad, she could not keep up the fast. She was confused on what to do next since she has failed at the warrior diet. She was advised by a friend and co-worker of hers that it is advisable for her to go see a dietician in order to know which one suits her. She later went to the dietician and she was told that she has to start little by little.

The intermittent fasting process can be likened to the experience of a little boy and a bicycle. The boy had to go to the places he wanted to go like visiting friends on his foot. This was quite tiring to him. Then, he got a bicycle; this to him was the end of all his troubles. He decided to take his bicycle out one day and while going, he fell.

This was discouraging to him; he decided not to ride the bicycle ever again. Little did he know that to ride it is not easy? You will fall down a lot of times and by the time you get it, doing it will be very easy. You even close your eyes while riding it, and then you develop a lot of skills.

The intermittent fasting is not an easy scheme at first but this is due to your naivety to the scheme. After you finish learning about the skills, you will become an expert and could even teach other people encouraging them to never give up. To learn a bicycle would make you fall a lot of times but that is why I am here. To guide you through your challenge in order not to fall because most times, such falls could be very dangerous.

As a beginner in this program, try not to outdo yourself. Remember that you are new to the system, so is your body. Start little by little. It is most advisable to start with the 16/8 method or the spontaneous method. You could even form your own schedule. For example, let us say I am a accounts officer. This means I have to leave early in the morning. I could take a cup of coffee in the morning before going to work. Take some fruits and vegetables along in order to keep me sustained. When I get back in the evening, I will eat and this window would stop by 8-9 pm. The cycle continues. I can also decide to not take anything at all except water until I get back and eat my dinner. All depends on your schedule, work and most importantly your body. It is advisable to see a doctor before you start. This will let you know if you are fit to go or not. You should not disobey or disregard whatever the doctor says because if you do, it is highly detrimental to your health and life.

After some weeks, you will see that it is an easy thing to do because by then, you have gotten used to the system and you can now increase the hours by which you fast or change your approach to it in order to get more desired results.

Why not start today and see the goodness in intermittent fasting. Do not rush yourself all because you want to get a quick result. Take it slowly, as the saying goes, *"The journey of a thousand miles begins with a step."*

Choosing The Perfect Ketogenic Diet

The thought of having to make a choice most times puts most of us under pressure. I know it must be quite a task to choose the form of ketogenic diet you will do because of you want results and you would not want to partake in a type that does not bring out the desired result that you want. That is why I am here to guide you through and help you in choosing the perfect ketogenic diet. As I have mentioned earlier, the ketogenic diet has several approaches which include:

1] The Standard Ketogenic diet
2] The Targeted ketogenic diet
3] The Cyclic ketogenic diet
4] The High Protein ketogenic diet
5] The Protein Sparing Modified Fast

I am going to be explaining what each of them entails, the requirements, the rules and the type of people that it is most suitable for.

THE STANDARD KETOGENIC DIET

This is probably the most basic form of the ketogenic diet. It is used by most people who engage in the ketogenic diet. It entails the taking in of 50 grams of carbohydrate or less. This intake helps you to stay in the state of ketosis and it has been tested and trusted with the testimonies of people backing it up. The standard ketogenic diet is mostly used by the people who are new to the diet. It is meant for rapid weight loss, it is for people who desire to keep fit and lose weight. So, if you are almost obese or you are feeling that you have gained excess weight of recent. This is the best for you. It is quite easy; your energy supply would be coming from the proteins and fats that you eat. What it requires is just a drastic reduction in the of calories and carbohydrates you take in. It requires you to increase the number of fats you eat: this will supplement the energy supply that is being brought by carbohydrates.

If you are an office worker, this is the best for you. It works without stress.

THE TARGETED KETOGENIC DIET

If you love working out or exercising, then I think you might want to see this. The targeted ketogenic diet gives way for you to consume 30-50 grams of carbohydrates in a day. You might be wondering how you would burn the calories. It is quite simple. The TKD is mainly for people who work out and exercise, so the calories are burned during the workouts. The intake of the carbohydrate can be immediately before your workout or immediately after your workout. Calories are burn during workouts and exercise.

If you do not like to work out or exercise, this is really not for you. It can be that you are too busy to work out or go to the gym; this is not for you either. So, if your job is time-consuming, you are not advised to take on this approach to ketosis. If you have time on your schedule to spare, then this is designed for you.

There was a story of a woman. She exercises a lot but after her marriage, she lost it. She gained a lot of weight and could not keep fit again. She was about to go out to look for a job but she is afraid that she might not be accepted because of her body size. I would recommend this to her because not only will she lose weight and get a job but she would also be able to go back to her former hobby of exercising which has been said to keep the doctor away. So, to my exercise lovers: this is for you.

THE CYCLIC KETOGENIC DIET

As you already know, the ketogenic diet is not only known for the reduction of weight. It also treats other disorders like high blood pressure, heart disease, cancer, fatty liver and so on. This form of ketogenic diet is solely for athletes.

It is for professional athletes whose sports require a lot of energy like weight lifters, endurance runners, footballers and so on. If you are not one of these, it is not for you.

So, do not try it, else you would not see the desired results. The cyclic ketogenic diet requires a high level of carbohydrate consumption but these carbohydrates are later burned up during their sports activities. They would consume a high level of carbohydrate for two days before their competition in order to fully reload their glycogen storage. This will really help them in their muscle growth and also their power, although it can also lead to fat storage. This will really help in mental alertness, cognitive development and as said above improvement in muscle growth and power.

This is mainly for higher athletes. If you are not one: do not try it because if you do, you will not be able to burn up such amount of carbohydrate and therefore instead of losing weight, you are actually gaining more weight.

THE HIGH PROTEIN KETOGENIC DIET

This approach to ketogenic diet is for people that want to shed excess fats. That is, if you are overweight or obese, this is the perfect diet for you. The aim of this diet is to remove excess fat from the body and the removal of excess fat storage. This requires a high protein diet and through this high protein the excess fats are shed and it keeps the muscle mass lean. It builds the muscle mass in case you want to work out and it also sheds the excess fat that is already stored in the body. What is surprising is that it does not only shed the excess fats in the body but also uses it as a means of energy. While doing this, you will have to consume 1.5 grams of protein per muscle mass. This form of diet helps you to burn fats faster. While losing fats, it maintains your strength and energy levels.

This diet is for people who want a fast result in order to reach their fitness goals. It is more like the standard ketogenic diet; it is just that the proteins are higher.

So, if you are obese, it is advisable you try this out and you will see the difference.

THE PROTEIN SPARING MODIFIED FAST

This is a highly restrictive modification of the ketogenic diet. It includes mainly lean proteins and it is kept to 600-1000 calories a day. It is designed as a temporary solution to kick-start weight loss while preserving the muscle mass. Those that are on it avoid meat that is essentially higher in fat. Do not add fat while cooking and continue to avoid carbohydrate. The fat that produces the ketone bodies comes mainly from the fats that are stored up in the body. This model is a great temporarily; it is not sustainable to go as a lifestyle to its users.

This diet is quite promising in light of people who are really overweight. The diet serves as a kind of head start into the weight reduction scheme. But it is not really advisable to go for a long-term kind of lifestyle.

Above are various approaches to the ketogenic diet. There are various requirements and instructions to follow. All you have to do is to imagine yourself in each of the approaches and see which of them fits your best wishes regarding your fitness goals. Also look out for the one that suits your schedule and work the most. It is best advised to see a doctor or a dietician in order to avoid repercussions regarding your health and well being. All have been laid down for you, choose one today and your life will never remain the same.

Chapter Nine: What To Eat And Not To Eat

It should not be a surprise to you seeing people who took the ketogenic diet but there was still no improvement, or after there was an improvement, they went back to their former self.

Do not be surprised because the reason for that is their ignorance or their unwillingness to follow the instructions on what to eat and what not to eat.

There have been many speculations going all around the internet that one does not need to follow any rules; you are free to do anything as long as you are doing the ketogenic diet. This is a blatant lie and unconfirmed rumor. Some of these were treated when we were talking about the various misconceptions regarding the ketogenic diet.

The feeling of freedom comes to mind when you start to see the wonderful effects of the ketogenic diet but these actions we carry out during or after the program affects the results we will see and this can be discouraging.

I am here to tell you the things you should do and things that you should not do at all during your ketogenic diet challenge.

WATCH THE FATS YOU EAT

This is one of the things you need to watch out for during your ketogenic diet challenge. You must extensively watch the type of fats you put in your system. Since the fats entail 80% of your meals, is it not worth watching?

DRINK A LOT OF WATER

It is advised by doctors and health professionals that staying hydrated during the diet helps in your weight reduction goals. Staying hydrated is key in achieving your fitness goals.

ALCOHOL INTAKE

The matter of alcohol intake has been a controversial one by many scholars and professionals. It has been said that alcohol should not be taken during the ketogenic diet. This is due to the carbohydrate concentration in most of the wines and beers, but not all. Some types of alcohol are actually carbohydrate free and that means that they are keto friendly. What should be watched is the way you consume it. Although, it has been shown that the ketogenic diet increases the resistance one has to alcohol.

JUNK AND LATE NIGHT SNACK

This is one of the things that you should step away from. I know that it is quite hard to keep away from these things because when we were lonely and no one was there for us, they kept us comfortable and feeling wanted.

But these things are what led to you to start doing the ketogenic diet. Most of the time you look into the mirror, you do not like what you see due to your excess weight and these are the things that caused the excess fat.

So, indirectly, you hate them, you just do not know it yet. This junk food is detrimental to your health and can debar you from reaching your fitness goals.

On the long run, they cause diabetes, high blood sugar level, kidney problems, liver diseases, and most of all, obesity, and this is what you are trying to prevent.

So eating junk is likened to you shooting yourself in the leg. The issue of midnight snacks is common to most of us. Sometimes, we just want to treat ourselves to a late night snack of chicken, potato chips, ice cream, chocolates, burger, and pizza and so on. This can be due to a hard day's work or you doing something spectacular and you decided to appreciate yourself. This is really bad and it affects your body system. You might be wondering how. Let me explain to you.

The body system has a time it is active and has time to rest. It has been said that the digestive system rests from 10pm-4am. So taking a midnight snack is not only taking the risk of indigestion but also wearing out your body organs because they have no time to rest. It can be tempting and will not be easy to drop, but look at it as a stumbling block to achieving your fitness goals. It is not an advice but a must that you stop late night snacking and eating junk. Abiding by this will hasten the rate at which you lose weight.

THINGS TO DO AND THINGS NOT TO DO

DO EXERCISE WHEN OPPORTUNE

If you are the exercising type, it is fully advised to exercise alongside your ketogenic diet challenge. There is a misconception that the ketogenic diet disallows the use of workouts during it. This is a blatant lie. The use of exercise while dieting helps in the restoration of your muscle mass, energy, and keeping fit.

In case your schedule does not allow you to go to the gym or exercise, it is not necessarily important to get into the gym. If you cannot get into the gym, you can also buy workout DVD that you can use in your house.

DO WATCH YOUR CALORIES

This is very important to the successful completion of your ketogenic diet challenge. Try to watch the number of calories that you take in because too much of it will not only ruin your results but also store up in your body system, which will lead you to gain more weight instead of losing it. So watch your calorie intake in order to get the desired result.

DO AVOID FAST FOOD

For the fact that you can easily get burgers in a fast food restaurant is not really healthy. The foods are filled with chemicals and preservatives. Most of the time, they do not use cheese that is real. Even the salad might have hidden sugar sometimes.

DO not search for information about something after you might have finished eating it. Search for the information before you start eating it.

Chapter Ten: Tips On Ketogenic Diet

I will be giving you some tips that will help you with your ketogenic diet challenge. The tips are kind of shortcuts to having a successful ketogenic diet.

CLEAR CARBOHYDRATES FROM YOUR KITCHEN

Most people will only stick to the ketogenic diet if they had access to healthy ketogenic foods. This will help you a lot in avoiding falling prey to the carbohydrate concentrated foods in your cabinet. Clean your kitchen from high-carbohydrate foods like pastry, bread, potatoes, soda, rice, and candy. This will help a long way in achieving the ketogenic diet.

HAVE KETOGENIC SNACKS AT HAND

Having to prepare a lot of homemade meals is a big challenge for people as regards the ketogenic diet. There is a solution for you: why not have ketogenic snacks instead whenever you are hungry and you are not at home?

You can buy ketogenic snacks like hard boiled eggs, beef jerky, pre-cooked bacon, pre-made guacamole and so on or you can have them on the go. You can prepare a lot of them and this will not allow you to buy carbohydrate-heavy snacks.

BUY A FOOD SCALE

This might sound surprising but it is quite crucial. As it has been said, *"Drops of water make an ocean."* The amount of food you eat matters even to the tiniest form. Buy a food scale to measure your food and make sure you are eating the appropriate size because even the least can make a difference.

For example, 2 extra tablespoons of almond butter turn out to be an additional 200 calories and 6 grams of carbohydrates. It is not necessary you use the food scale till the end of your challenge. It is just for you to get the appropriate measurement then you can eyeball to measure it as you continue.

EXERCISE FREQUENTLY

I have mentioned a lot. Exercising allows your body to break down the glycogen it has in store. It also helps you to get fit and healthy. It also helps you in maintaining your muscle mass and strengthens you.

TRY INTERMITTENT FASTING

This is one of the most effective tips that can get you right on track to achieving your fitness goals. It helps you get into ketosis and lose weight. This means that you do not eat anything that contains calories for a given period of time. A study in Harvard has made it known that intermittent fasting manipulates your mitochondria in a way that the ketogenic diet also does and this elongates your lifespan. When you stop taking calories for some time, your body will start breaking down the excess glucose in your body obtained from consuming carbohydrates.

INCLUDE COCONUT OIL INTO YOUR DIET

Coconut oil contains fats called medium chain triglycerides which help you to quickly get into ketosis. Unlike other fats, the MCTs get quickly absorbed into the liver where they can be used for energy or they can be converted into ketones.

Frequently Asked Questions And Answers To Them

I will be answering frequently asked questions regarding the ketogenic diet.

Can pregnant women do the ketogenic diet?

The ketogenic has appeared safe due to the women that have done it and the doctors that have administered it to their patients during pregnancy. I cannot say I am right because there is no scientific research or study that has proved this. So, there is a lack of knowledge concerning this. The ketogenic diet may be very helpful in case of gestational diabetes. It is therefore advised that caution is to be exercised for a ketogenic diet during pregnancy unless there is a benefit you want to achieve while doing it in your own case.

At what level should my ketones be during ketosis?

Your ketones should be above 0.5mmol/l and this is general.

Can I develop muscles while doing my ketogenic diet?

Sure! It is even advised to do so but it is not compulsory. You can do this by going to the gym to work out; you can even buy the workout DVD if you do not have the time to go to the gym. Like I said earlier, it is not compulsory.

How long can I be on the ketogenic diet?

As long as you want! That is why the ketogenic diet is often referred to as a lifestyle. You can do it as long as you desire.

How long does it take to be in ketosis?

This is a popular question among those who are just starting the ketogenic diet. It actually varies from two weeks or more. People with more insulin resistance usually take a longer time before they get to ketosis. Lean and young people usually get to ketosis faster.

Conclusion

This brings us to the end of our book. I know you have in one way or the other derived and gotten the perfect tools to help you go through your ketogenic diet challenge.

It is not that easy. It is like driving a car: at first, it is very hard to comprehend and the fear of crashing comes to mind. Then when you start driving, the road seems confusing. This book will serve as a tool you will use to perfectly know how to drive through the odds and get to the finish line.

When you start learning how to drive, you won't immediately know how to overtake, change lanes, and the uses of the devices in the car, how to reverse, and even to hit the horn. Everything is one after the other. Like I said earlier, *"the journey of a thousand miles begins with a step."* It is one step after the other and this book will help and guide you through this journey.

It has been a great pleasure for us to impart and flash the torch which points out the way to you. We are delighted that this book of ours has been a tool in modifying your life and taking you across the finish line of that journey of a thousand miles.

The ketogenic diet, if not the best, is one of the best ways in reducing body weight and excess fat. It was designed for the treatment of seizures, but unknown to mankind; it is like an onion of blessings. Within it, there are a lot of benefits and layers of treatment. It has been tested and trusted by many scientists all over the world.

Make sure you visit your doctor for you to be fit for this amazing treasure because an expert's point of view is also needed.

Thank you for reading our book today and make sure you also share this great treasure to everyone around because with this the world can be a better place. Let the ketogenic diet be a part of you because the ketogenic diet is not a diet, it is a lifestyle!

Show the world the lifestyle!

Intermittent Fasting For Women:

The Powerful Secret For Women Who Want To Lose Weight With Ketogenic Diet, Heal Your Body Through intermittent process and Live Healthy with Meal Plan.
By: Amy Moore

Table of Contents

Introduction
Chapter 1: What Is Fasting?
Chapter 2: What Is the Ketogenic Diet and How It Works with Intermittent Fasting?
Chapter 3: Different Fasting Methods
Chapter 4: Fasting Tips and FAQs
Chapter 5: Fasting Recipes

    Breakfast
    Baked Eggs
    Breakfast Salad
    Breakfast Patties
    Avocado Zucchini
    Simple Chia Pudding
    Lunch
    Cauliflower Nachos with Turkey Meat
    Skirt Steak with Red Pepper
    Easy Tomato Soup
    Salmon, Avocado, and Sweet Kale Salad with a Lemon Vinaigrette
    Halibut and Lemon Pesto
    Dinner
    Cold Cucumber Soup
    Caprese Tomato Salad
    Grilled Cabbage Steaks
    Roasted Chicken and Zucchini in One Pan
    Portobello Pizza
    Snacks
    Mini Zucchini Pizzas
    Spinach and Turkey Pinwheels
    Broccoli Salad with Bacon

Cauliflower Hummus
Linseed or Flax Seed Crackers

Conclusion

Introduction

Congratulations on downloading *Intermittent Fasting: The Beginner's Guide for Women Who Want to Lose Weight with The Ketogenic Diet for Ultimate Weight-Loss and Fat Burning*, and thank you for doing so.

There is something that must have sparked your interest in intermittent fasting, and I hope that I can give insight into why intermittent fasting is a lifestyle that anyone can and should do.

There are lots of people who struggle with their weight. They jump back and forth between fad diet after fad diet seeing limited to no results. Some people may go to the gym one week and the weeks do not go at all. They have no motivation or desire to be healthy. Other people are so busy with their families and careers that they do not have time to give attention to their health, especially their diet. These people pick up fast food on the way to work and on the way home, and their bodies are taking a major hit. Other people are interested in being healthy but have no idea where to begin. Everyone knows that you should prioritize your health, but if you have never been talked or seen healthy habits practiced, they run around like a chicken with its head cut off. Feeling discouraged about not knowing where to begin their health (if they even care at all), all of these people just give up and succumb to a lifestyle of unhealthy eating and unhealthy habits. All of us have been one of these people in life. Maybe you are one of these people who has hit rock bottom, and you know that you have to do something about your health or you will suffer dire consequences. Look no further; the solution you are looking for is on the way.

There is a way for you to get your weight under control and to be the healthy person that you know you can be. This method also works for people who are already healthy as well. The easiest way to get healthy is to gain control of your diet. If you can control your diet, gaining or losing weight becomes a lot easier. Even for those who have had to struggle with their diet, there is help. The easiest way to get your diet under control is by intermittent fasting. Intermittent fasting is all about limiting the time that you eat, with a focus on eating healthy foods when you do eat. Ultimately, intermittent fasting helps you maintain healthy portion control and lends itself to an overall improvement in one's health. It helps you fight sugar cravings and unsavory inflammatory illnesses that can hinder one for life.

Intermittent fasting is easy, simple, and a relatively painless way to lead a healthier lifestyle. Once you understand the basic principles, you can find ways to incorporate the changes within your lifestyle for maximum health gains. With this book, there are no longer any excuses that will hinder you from committing to this lifestyle. Everything you need to begin and sustain intermittent fasting is laid out for you plainly and simply in this book. This book is grateful to be a part of your transformation and commitment to a healthier lifestyle. Thank you for making a commitment to yourself and to the people who care about you. By the time you finish reading, you'll be able to discuss intermittent fasting with ease and conviction as a proud practitioner.

The following chapters will discuss everything you need to know about fasting. Chapter 1 explores what fasting is and why it is good for you. Chapter 2 explains how to intermittent fast and how to use the ketogenic diet while fasting. Different fasting methods are discussed in Chapter 3, and Chapter 4 gives fasting tips and answers to frequently asked questions about fasting. Chapter 5 gives you a few easy ketogenic recipes that will help you start your intermittent fasting journey. Be sure to take notes about the info that is most appealing to you. It will help you find it easier if you want to reference later. "Happy reading!" By the time you finish, I hope I can say, "Happy Fasting!"

There are plenty of books on this subject on the market, thanks again for choosing this one! Every effort was made to ensure it is full of as much useful information as possible, please enjoy!

Chapter 1: What Is Fasting?

Why would one be interested in fasting? Why would someone forego their favorite foods in order to get healthier? This chapter will explain everything fasting and show you the advantages fasting can have in your life. Fasting has been important to many cultures all around the world. This chapter will give a brief overview of what fasting is, a short history, and end with the many benefits it has for people who want to lose weight, control type 2 diabetes, look younger, and improve their heart health. The chapter will end with a word of caution and give groups of people who should probably avoid fasting.

Fasting and starvation are often lumped together, but they are different. When a person starves, they do not have any food to eat, whereas, fasting is the purposeful foregoing of food. Starvation is out of person's control; a person does fasting in control. Lots of people reported mental clarity, ease with digestion issues, weight loss, easier sleeping, and a simpler, cleaner, more convenient way of eating as a few of the benefits of fasting. It is also important to note that intermittent fasting is not just a diet. It is a lifestyle change where you eat specifically during a set period of time, and you go without eating for another set period of time. Depending on the results you want, you can make the window of time when you eat bigger or the window of time when you do not eat bigger.

Fasting is as old as humankind itself. It has long been touted for its health benefits for the body and spiritual wellness. The benefits of fasting are hard-wired into our body as a biological mechanism against sickness. Think about the last time you were very sick. Did you want to eat? Of course not! As a matter of fact, when you ate, you probably wanted to throw up any of the food you ate. Hence, fasting is a biologic way to protect one's body when you are sick. Not only as an automatic biologic response to sickness, when you look into ancient history, but fasting was also a well-known remedy for illnesses. Greek philosophers often considered intermittent fasting as a solution to getting better. Ancient documents show many doctors prescribing fasting as a way to deal with illness. Despite the lack of modern tools, it is absolutely amazing how doctors knew that fasting and its different variations were a surefire way to deal with illnesses.

Additionally, fasting is a common solution to increase concentration or devoutness in the spiritual realm. Ezra Taft Benson, American politicians and religious leaders were right on the money when describing the mental and health benefits of intermittent fasting. Lots of religions practice some form of fasting as a way to connect with the Divine. Christians have fasted as a way to clean mental fogginess and realign their spiritual purpose. Muslims fast every year during Ramadan as a form of spiritual cleansing. Others have used fasting to make political statements which shows the power of fasting has on others as a show of solidarity for important issues that one believes in. Some cultures like Italians and other European countries usually have a heavy lunch and a light breakfast or dinner, which as a form of intermittent fasting. Italians are often lauded worldwide for their diet with many others trying to emulate it in their day-to-day life. As you can see, fasting has been everywhere and is an important part of the human experience.

What intermittent fasting superior to other dieting methods is that it is a lifestyle. Unlike following a diet for a short of time in order to see limited results, intermittent fasting is a lifestyle choice that one follows every day. The main purpose of a diet is often times to lose weight. However, with intermittent fasting losing weight is only one benefit of the intermittent fasting lifestyle. Intermittent fasting has numerous benefits with weight loss only being an extra. Intermittent fasting has been linked to improving mental health, chronic illness, and heart disease, even helping to prevent certain cancers and seizures. The lifestyle change and extended health benefits are what makes intermittent fasting superior to other diets and methods. The best thing about intermittent fasting is, once you get into the habit of doing it, the health results stay with you for years. You do not have to worry about getting into the horrible cycle of gaining weight and losing weight. Intermittent fasting is a habit that is inherently healthy and easier for one to maintain over long periods of time because it is something that you do every day without having to think about it. You can also mold it to fit the most hectic or most laid-back lifestyles.

While science is still studying all the benefits of intermittent fasting, the best thing about intermittent fasting is that ancient people already knew about the results. Whether to heal sickness or increase mental and spiritual well-being, intermittent fasting is a multi-tier approach to healing your entire body. Now is the time to touch base with the wisdom of our forefathers and get back to this lifestyle that has shown to be beneficial to our human ancestors and modern people alike. If you are looking for a way to improve your body and mind at the same time, then intermittent fasting is exactly what you are looking for to do so. If done correctly, it is as safe as other diet methods and has the potential to stick with you a lot longer than fad dieting.

There are many reasons that people decide to fast. The main draw for many is the potential to lose weight. Fasting does not just help you lose weight, but it helps you to lose weight in one of the most stubborn places - your stomach. How many of us have struggled to try to lose those love handles and that muffin top! Never fear, intermittent fasting is the solution that you've been looking for to tackle these spots. Because intermittent fasting inherently restricts your meals to a certain time, you are already lowering your daily caloric intake. When you do that, you end up losing weight. However, what makes intermittent fasting more effective is that fasting that causes your weight loss hormones to rev up. When you are in a fasted state, your body gets energy from your body's fat stores and not the food that you are eating. This, in turn, increasing your metabolism rate. So what is your metabolism rate? That is the rate at which you lose calories. You can lose calories by either eating less food or getting your body to use your stored fat, which is what intermittent fasting does — a definite win-win.

Additionally, intermittent fasting helps you not to lose that much muscle compared to just fasting. When you still have some type of muscle on your body, your muscles work harder than fat to increase your metabolism, so you are losing weight while doing limited activities. When your muscles are used to this time of method of eating, you are essentially eating your way to losing weight, which is extremely helpful in the long-term of trying to maintain a healthy weight and healthy lifestyle. Another hormone that is affected by intermittent fasting is leptin. This hormone tells your brain which then tells your body when you are hungry. If you are obese, this hormone is overactive. Your body reads this hunger cue no matter if you are hungry or not which cause you to overeat. Thus, the extra food and energy make you gain weight. When you fast, it helps improve your leptin sensitivity, so your body is more in tune with your hunger triggers, like ghrelin. Intermittent fasting sends your brain more measured indicators of your hunger, so you are not overeating. However, it is important to stick to a pattern of fasting, especially if you are intermittent fasting, to avoid an increase of cortisol, which can lead to more stress or insomnia if you are not consistent with your fasting window.

Another reason people fast is to control type 2 diabetes. Diabetes is a chronic illness that occurs when a person's body is not able to send glucose, or blood sugar to your body. Glucose is what your body eat and in order to get that glucose your body needs insulin. People with type 1 diabetes do not produce insulin at all. Whereas people with type 2 diabetes produce insulin, but their bodies don't use the insulin as efficiently as it should. As type 2 diabetes progresses, people tend not to make insulin at all. Dr. Jason Fung did a study where 3 men fasted for a time frame of 10 months. Two of the men fasted every other day. And one man fasted three days a week. On the days that the men fasted, they were able to have low-calorie drinks like coffee, tea, and water. They could also have one low-calorie meal.

At the end of the study, two of the men did not take any of their diabetes drugs. The last man had stopped taking four out of the five drugs that he was taking to control his diabetes. Dr. Fung asserts that fasting can be helpful for those with type 2 diabetes. However, other doctors caution against people taking this study as the complete truth since the study was only limited to three people.

Nevertheless, the results seem quite promising. The most important thing from this study was Dr. Jason Fung demonstrated that fasting does have a positive effect on controlling diabetes. In the future, fasting will most likely be used as an important way to regulate, if not cure, type 2 diabetes. An important consideration before fasting it to remember that if you are taking medication for your type 2 diabetes, you need to check in with your physician before attempting to fast to control your type 2 diabetes.

Another reason people choose to fast is to improve their physical appearance. Fasting reduces oxidative stress. To understand how oxidative stress works, there first must be a quick definition of what free radicals are. Free radicals are atoms in your body that are unstable. In order to get stable, the free radicals have to join two other substances in your body to get stable. When free radicals join with other substances in your body, it causes oxidative stress. Hence, oxidative stress can cause cells to break down in your body and can result in issues such as inflammation and wrinkles and diseases or even chronic diseases. When you fast, it helps your body prevent forming these free radicals that can destroy your body in so many ways. Intermittent fasting also increases the human growth hormone which increases your body's collagen production. More collagen means that your body will have younger-looking skin.

Moreover, fasting increases the process of autophagy, which is how your body repairs itself by making newer and healthier cells. When you have newer and healthier cells, your skin improves. Fasting also helps the fluid that accumulates under the skin lessen, which also improves your overall appearance since salt is eliminated from your body when you fast. Less salt in your body increases your appearance and slows down the aging process.

The last major benefit of fasting that will be explored in this chapter is when people fast to improve their heart health. High blood pressure, cholesterol, diabetes, and obesity are all indicators of heart health problems. Fasting helps reduce all of these risks. However, fasting can cause an imbalance of your electrolytes, so when a person fasts, they must make sure that they are consuming enough electrolytes to not affect their heart health negatively. More about electrolytes will be discussed later in the book.

Before the chapter ends, a word of caution must be given. Some people should not fast. Those include people that have a history of eating disorders, pregnant women, breastfeeding women, teenagers, children and those with type 1 diabetes. Those with chronic illness or even cancers should also consult with their doctors before fasting. The rule of thumb is to always consult with any health professional before you begin fasting. While it is great to have the desire to want to do intermittent fasting, before you begin, you will first want to check with your health professional before embarking on the fasting journey no matter if you are healthy or not. This is important to make sure you are fasting healthily and safely. Fasting should not make you feel sick. You will feel hunger, but if at any point, you begin to feel weird while fasting or run into any issues, keep an open line of communication open with your doctor or preferred health care provider.

Now that you know all the benefits and history of fasting, it's time to learn one of the best ways to see vast improvements with your intermittent fasting by coupling it with the keto diet! Turn the page to learn more.

Chapter 2: What Is the Ketogenic Diet and How It Works with Intermittent Fasting?

Intermittent fasting is when you simply avoid eating food for a certain period of time. There are many different methods of intermittent fasting you can choose from which will be explored in the next chapter. To improve the results people get from intermittent fasting, they decide to do the keto diet or a vegan or vegetarian diet. I'm sure you've heard about the keto diet. Now it's time to learn more about it.

What Is the Keto Diet?

The keto diet is a low carbohydrate diet that helps prevent certain diseases and helps a person lose weight. It has been known to help people manage their type 2 diabetes and in some cases their epilepsy. Some people choose to eliminate carbs altogether, while others limit their carbohydrate intake.

The main word in the keto diet is 'Keto.' Ketones are a type of fuel your body uses when your blood sugar or glucose, the type of sugar you get from carbohydrates like grains and starches are in short supply. Your body can make ketones when you eat a limited amount of carbs and a moderate amount of protein.

Your body can make ketones from fat; then your body can use the ketones for energy, especially your brain. Since our bodies are always working, our brain even more so, it needs energy. Our brain can run off glucose and ketones.

When a person is on the keto diet, they run on fat which helps them lose weight. When your body creates ketones, you enter ketosis which means your body is effectively burning fat most of the time. The easiest way to get to this state is by fasting.

Since a person is unable to fast all the time, using a keto diet helps you be in ketosis the majority of the time. Weight loss is not the only benefit of the keto diet. Many people benefit from the way the keto diet can help treat certain disease. Some of the diseases that the keto diet helps treat prevent or lower the risk factor of having to include the following.

- Parkinson's Disease- The keto diet hasn't shown to help improve the symptoms of this disease.
- Heart disease - The keto diet improves risk factors like blood sugar blood pressure HDL cholesterol levels in body fit which are can help a person improve their risk factors for heart disease.
- Acne – The keto diet improves your sugar intake can help a person improve and prevent acne.
- Brain injuries - After brain injuries in animal, that hell in recovery.
- Polycystic ovary syndrome - Since the keto diet reduces insulin levels, it has shown to help those with polycystic ovary syndrome.

How to Use the Keto Diet with Intermittent Fasting

When on the keto diet, you want to avoid the following foods.

- Sugar - This includes sugary drinks, desserts, junk foods, and snacks.
- Root tubers and vegetables - Carrots, sweet potatoes, potato, and parsnips.
- Fruit - Because of the high sugar content, you want to limit fruit.
- Sauces and condiments - Be on the lookout for certain sauces and condiments because I can contain unhealthy fat and sugar.
- Unhealthy fats - Try to avoid processed avoids and mayonnaise.
- Alcohol - Because alcohol contains a lot of carbohydrates,

you want to avoid them.

On the positive side, you can have lots of food while on the keto diet. Those foods include:

- Nuts and Seeds – Chia seeds, pumpkin seeds, flax seeds, walnuts, and almonds are all great to eat.
- Meat - Chicken, turkey, sausage, bacon are a few meats you can have.
- Fatty fish -Trout, mackerel, tuna, and salmon to name a few.
- Eggs - Have as many eggs as you want!
- Low carb veggies - Tomatoes, green veggies, peppers, and onions are all up for grabs!
- Healthy oils- Avocado and olive oil are great to have.

The great thing about the ketogenic diet is you can couple it with your intermittent fasting to get the results that you want. The next chapter will go into more detail about the different intermittent fasting methods you can have with the keto diet.

Chapter 3: Different Fasting Methods

Now that we have discusses the background of fasting, it's now important to offer practical advice about getting started. This chapter is dedicated to giving you tips that can help you deal with your hunger and survive the fasting process. Attention will be given to different fasts that are possible, including intermittent and other fasts. We will end with a list of fluids that you must have in order to deal with fasting long-term. To begin the process, there are three steps that you can take to get started.

Some people think that you need a lot of time and a big budget to get started intermittent fasting. The truth is that you don't need any of those things. You just need the determination and willpower to begin. Essentially, you can get started with 3 easy steps.

1- Choose which fasting method you want to follow. – There are lots of different methods of fasting you can select from. Once you choose one, stick to it and begin the process. Do not feel obligated to continue a fasting method if you know that your body is responding negatively. You can always select a different method to follow.

2- Calculate your calories and make sure you have a well-balanced diet. Create a meal plan. Decide if you want to be vegetarian or vegan for more intense results. Do not underestimate the importance of counting your calories. Taking the time to plan your meals and make sure your calories are not going over your daily caloric count or under by too much will be the difference to being able to intermittent fasting correctly or not. Some people eat too much or too little. Do not be that person who fasts, but is still unhealthy.

3- Decide which exercise you want to follow on the days that you are not fasting. – If you are going to exercise while fasting, make sure that you choose methods that are conducive to your fasting days. Take it easy on the days that you are fasting and go harder on the days that you are not fasting. If you need a little extra boost for the days you work out, try carbohydrate loading which is bulking up your meals with carbohydrates to help you make it through your workout. For longer fasts, do not worry about trying to exercise while fasting.

The rest of the book will go into more details about these three different steps. Feel free to take notes so you can come back and read your highlighted info. Don't feel pressure to immediately be perfect from day one. This lifestyle is a process, and you can slowly acclimate yourself to it. When you put unnecessary pressure on yourself, you add unneeded stress which can delay or hamper your results. Remember this is supposed to be fun and it's supposed to be about being a healthier person. Staying happy and positive will ensure that you will be fasting for years to come.

Choose Your Intermittent Fasting Method

Now, what about all those fasting methods we keep talking about? We'll begin talking about intermittent fasting first. Intermittent fasting is eating during certain windows and then not eating during other windows. It may sound complicated, but it's really not. Most people have done some sort of fasting without even knowing. The easiest way to practice intermittent fasting is to skip the meal that is easiest for you according to your current schedule. This version is called spontaneous fasting. Maybe you are in a rush and forget to eat breakfast. You just intermittently fasted! Perhaps you are preparing for a busy meeting and decide to skip lunch. Yup, you just intermittently fasted. Spontaneous intermittent fasting is very easy to do, and many often partake in it without knowing it. To make this method more effective, instead of missing a meal by accident, you will miss it purposefully. If you are already doing this accidentally, then you can just fine tune it so it can become your official intermittent fasting method. This is definitely one of the easiest methods to do since it happens without you thinking about it. However, there are other methods that you can definitely consider, as well.

The next version of intermittent fasting is called The Warrior Diet. When you practice this version of intermittent fasting, you only eat small pieces of raw fruits and vegetables during the day and eat one major meal at night. The major meal you eat should be limited to about 500-600 calories for women and 800-900 calories for men. Muslims practice a form of this intermittent fasting version during Ramadan when they forgo eating during the day and only eat after sunset.

Every other day fasting is when you fast every other day. During this version of fasting, you eat a limited amount of meals during your off days and on the days that you are allowed to eat you just eat regularly. A similar version of this intermittent fasting method is called the 5:2. During this method, you eat for 5 full days, and you fast for 2 days by only eating a total of 500 to 600 calories on the days that you are fasting. For women, if you are using this method, it is advised that you eat 500 calories, and for men, it is advised that you eat 600 calories. You can break your smaller meals into two meals of 300 calories or 250 calories respectively. The trick when using this method is to eat the same amount as you would if you were eating regularly on the days that you can eat. You also do not want to fast for two days in a row, especially for women. It is advised that you break up the fasting days during the week so that the two fasting days are not one after the other. With this intermittent fasting method, it is extremely important to meal plan to make sure that you are reaching your caloric limit. This method requires that you are vigilant about your meal planning so that you are not overeating or undereating. This method can definitely be more challenging to start with, but once you get into the habit of doing it, it will become a lot easier.

One of the most popular versions of intermittent fasting is called the 16/8 fast. While you do this type of fast, you only eat during an 8 to 10-hour window and then you fast the other 16 hours of the day. Popular times to fast can be from 10 am to 6 pm, or 9 am to 5 pm, or even 11 am to 7 pm. This method of fasting is beneficial because you are able to follow your natural hunger cycles. Some people are never hungry in the morning, so they are able to forgo breakfast. Some people do not like to eat after a certain amount of time in the evening, so they forego dinner. By using this method of fasting, you are able to add intermittent fasting to your lifestyle without having to make a major adjustment. To take this method to the next level, some people fast for 20 hours and only eat during a 4-hour window.

The more you fast, the more you can potentially lose weight as long as you are making sure that you are eating healthy during your eating times. One of the most difficult intermittent fasting methods is called the 24-hour fast. Some people fast from dinner one day to the end of the next day or breakfast one day to breakfast the next day. For beginners, it is probably best to start off with a smaller window and work your way up to not eating for longer periods of time. Only the most advanced, most determined fasters should try this initially. This method also requires lots of willpower and self-control. People who are new to intermittent fasting my read this and think, 'Who in the world is trying this method of intermittent fasting?' Sure, actors and actresses may use this method to get ready for movie roles, but a lot of regular people use it, too. You will be surprised that it is very convenient for lots of people to follow. As you become more versed with intermittent fasting, you may find that you too that prefer The Warrior Diet over different methods of intermittent fasting.

Another popular intermittent fasting, one that has the most research done on it, is the every other day fast, or alternate daily fasting (ADF). Don't let the name fool you. Alternate daily fasting is similar to the 5:2 diet in that you can eat up to 500 calories on the days that you fast. The only difference is that you fast on alternate days than 2 times a week like in the 5:2 diets. Intermittent fasting is usually less than 24 hours, but there are those who have had smashing success with longer diets, specifically, 24-hour, 36-hour, 42-hour and 2-week fasts.

If at some point you feel comfortable with intermittent fasts, you can consider moving to extended fasts, starting with at least 24-hours.

Before you begin an extended fast, make sure you have consulted with a medical professional and are comfortable with your reasons for partaking upon the fast. Once you have this figured out, you will be able to move to prepare for the fast. You should know that extended fasting is perfectly safe and will cause you to reevaluate how you think of hunger. By the time you finish with your extended fast, you will no longer think of hunger as a negative. Daresay, you may think of it as a way to improve your mental health. And accept hunger for what it is – a brief moment that you can master. When you decide to do an extended fast, do not be afraid hunger, rather figure out ways to master it.

A 24-hour fast

One of the easiest ways to break into a longer fasting period is to start with a 24-hour fast. A 24 hour fast is great for giving your physical body a reset. It helps reset your system for issues related to your appetite, gut, and energy. When you begin this fast, you want to still go through your regular routine. When your fasting for 24 hours or longer, try to stay away from food so you won't be tempted and try to keep your mind clear from thinking about food. Remember, anyone can fast up to three days without any medical supervision. If you are doing an alternate day fast or a 5:2 fast, you can slowly transition to going to one full day of not eating.

The night before you begin your fast is very important, so make sure that you are eating a balanced meal. Get up and start your day like normal. You can even start off with tea or water or coffee. And go through your regular activities. By the time you finish, you will notice that your 24 hours have gone by quickly. Once it's time to break the fast, don't just eat a huge meal. Slowly ease into the meal, so you don't get sick. Start off by drinking a nice warm glass of lemon water that will prepare your stomach for the coming meal. Wait thirty minutes and then have a low carb snack. Wait another thirty minutes and then eat a nice, well-balanced meal. Also, don't overdo the meal. After any fast, do not eat everything you see to avoid gaining unnecessary weight. Control your urges so you can get the most out of your fast. Also, don't be alarmed if you have to go to the bathroom more after you fast. It's your body's natural reaction to your higher metabolism that may occur after a fast. You can take a probiotic before eating to try and regulate your urge.

A 36-hour fast

A 36-hour fast is extremely helpful for those who have type 2 diabetes due to their higher insulin resistance compared to those with type 1 diabetes. For this type of fast, it is recommended that a person does it 2-3 times a week for those with type 2 diabetes. People who don't have diabetes will also benefit from this fast. One of the easiest ways to do it is to have dinner around 6 or 7 pm on Day 1. On Day 2, you wouldn't eat any meals, only drink fluids with no calories added. Then you wouldn't eat until 6 or 7 am on the third day. It may feel weird at first, but this type of fast is definitely doable.

A 42-hour fast

A 42-hour fast builds on the 36-hour fast. You would still have dinner around 6 pm on Day 1. On Day 2, you wouldn't eat any meals, only drink fluids with no calories added. Then you wouldn't eat until noon on the third day. An easy way to transition into a 42-hour fast is to get into the habit of having your first meal around noon-time. To start this habit, in the morning, you would wake up and have a cup of coffee or water. If you get into the habit of having your first meal around noon, your body won't feel as hungry when you first wake up.

It is important to remember than when you are doing a longer fast. You don't want to restrict your calories. Eat normal sized meals, but don't overdo it. You may think that you will want to eat everything in sight once you finish your fast, but you may realize that your appetite goes down. So eating until you are full does not result in a huge feast like expected.

A two-week fast

A two-weeks fasting protocol builds on all the other fasts. It's essentially a water fast for 2 weeks. Before beginning this type of fast; you want to prepare. Before you begin, take the time to detox from unhealthy foods and habits like smoking and not getting enough sleep. Food you will want to avoid include dairy, sugar, alcohol, eggs, fish, caffeinated drinks and meat. Try to eat raw foods every day for about a week before to make the longer fat easier to maintain.

After you have prepared, you can start the time to fast. You may be hungry but resist the urge to eat. The desire for hunger normally passes after three days. Stay hydrated to help you get through this stage. It's at this stage that people begin to think clearer and feel empowered. While staying hydrated, you also want to make sure you are taking your electrolytes. You can take them via supplements. You'll want to have magnesium, phosphate, calcium, potassium, and sodium. You will want to check with your preferred medical provider before embarking upon such a fast. A two-week can go fast quickly, and you can trigger fatal symports if you are not prepared properly. You may also experience extreme mood swings, so give your friends and family the heads up.

As you get deeper into the fast, you will start to feel fatigued, even dizziness, and sometimes blurred vision. Your breath can smell bad, and you may even get sick. This is your body's detox process. It shows that your body is responding well to the fast by getting rid of the toxins in your body. You may even experience some flu-like symptoms, like pains, aches, chills, and fevers. This is just your body's way of getting rid of the toxins by pushing them through your intestines, skins, lungs, nose, and stomach.

As some point, you will overcome the plateau. You will feel normal. You may even go back in forth between feeling sick and feeling normal. Again, this is your body responding positively to the fast. Stick it out if you can. If you notice any of the extreme symptoms from earlier in the book, that's when you want to reach out to your medical provider. If you can make it through a 2-week fast, you will feel amazed afterward.

For this type of fast, do not try to workout - just take it easy. Be thoughtful and meditate. To make it through the fast, you can stay in airy and bright rooms. When you fast, your body may give off an odor, so this will help the odor dissipate quicker. The bright room will improve your mood. Also, try to take in the sun for about 10 to 20 minutes daily before it gets too hot. To help with your breath, brush your tongue with activated charcoal powder. You can also scrub your skin with a dry brush and bathe multiple times a day to keep the odor at bay. To take the fast to another level, you can take two enemas daily during the first week and only once until the fast is over. One of the most important things is to surround yourself with people who care if you're going to make it. They will help you get through the tough times.

When it's time to break the fast, go extremely slow. The longer you go without food, the longer you need to spend slowly reintroducing the food back into your life. You can start with bone broth and then small meals. Don't try to eat everything at once. Go slowly. Most people prefer intermittent fasting, but a longer fast has immense health and spiritual or mental benefits. Ultimately, it's up to you to decide if an extended fast is best for you or not.

Once you have figured out which fasting method you want to choose, the next thing you need to do before you begin intermittent fasting is to determine why you want to begin in the first place. What is your why? Why is it so important for you to start intermittent fasting? This can be a number of different reasons. Are you doing intermittent fasting in order to lose weight? Are you doing intermittent fasting to lead a healthier lifestyle? Are you doing intermittent fasting for another specific health outcome, like to lower your blood pressure or cholesterol levels or to even increase your metabolism or energy? Whatever your reason is before beginning, make that reason clear so you can always come back to it as a point of reference when you feel like you are getting weak at any moment.

While your weight loss and health journey is different than other people's, it is interesting to look at other people who fast to see what they're doing and what works for them. You can use them as inspiration. You can also form your own support group to hold you accountable for your reasons for intermittent fasting. You can find this support group online or in person, like a family member or trusted friend. Checking out online boards every now and then is also great to do in order to keep your info up-to-date and to recharger your intermittent fasting battery. If you are unable to find such a support group around, don't be afraid to start your own. Imagine how fun it will be to have a group of people supporting each other and knowing that you started it. People tend to be social and love to work out in groups. And intermittent fasting group can be a unique way to encourage yourself and encourage others and help a group of people get healthy at the same time. Popular places to look for people interested in such a group would be Craigslist, meetup.com, or even putting flyers in local coffee shops, doctor's offices or the library. Don't be shy if there isn't a group. It may be a sign that you are the one that is needed to start such a group.

The next thing you want to do before you begin is to speak with your doctor. When you meet, let your doctor know what your reasons for wanting to do intermittent fasting are. Then see if they have any input. This especially important if you have diabetes, are elderly or pregnant or have a history of eating disorders. If you fall into any of these categories, do not skip this step. The doctor can give you certain steps to avoid as well as give you some tips on how to take your results to the next level. Keeping your doctor aware of what you're doing can make sure that you always have a health professional in your corner and support to give you insight when you need it.

The next important step you should do before you begin is to have realistic expectations. If you plan on losing 50 pounds in a week, that's most likely not going to happen. It is healthy to lose at least two pounds a week. Even if you have a realistic expectation of how much weight you want to lose, what happens if you are not seeing the results you think you should be seeing? (We'll talk about this some in the next chapter.) The most important point about your expectations is to adjust them. You may not meet your expectations, and that is ok. You can adjust your expectations or adjust your actions to meet them. Do not get discouraged if you do not meet your expectations. Keep going! You do not want to throw in the towel too soon or throw the towel in without adjusting your expectations. No matter what your expectations are, continue to arm yourself with the proper information by researching so, you can see how intermittent fasting best fits into your lifestyle. When you have your reasons for doing intermittent fasting and your food journal ready, you can go ahead and begin.

Schedule your Day of Reckoning. This is the day where you get rid of everything in your kitchen that's not going to help you with your intermittent fasting journey. These items are things like junk food, alcohol, snacks, salty and sugary drinks. Sugary drinks include diet drinks and health drinks like Gatorade or Powerade. These all contain fructose which is just as deadly and inflammation causing as sugar. You can give those bad foods to a friend or family member, a food bank or just throw them away. For the more dramatic people like me, you can even burn them. This day of reckoning is a special day in your intermittent fasting journey. It is the day of no return, and it can symbolically signify your new lifestyle is an intermittent faster. This step can be as fun or as dramatic as you would like it. However, once you choose this day stick with it, so you know, it's time to begin a new way of life.

The next thing is, like Nike, 'Just do it!' Pick your fasting window and eating time and start. Initially, do not expect to just go 24 hours without food, definitely build up to that goal. When you start off slow, you can try to maybe just to avoid eating breakfast since you already sleeping and coming from a fast. Another way to get a slow start is if you try to reduce the portions of a certain food that you are eating before you totally give up the food that you are eating. For example, if you just have to have 10 cokes a day. Trying have 5 then 3 then 1 until you are at zero. Other ways to go incrementally fast are to perhaps change the portion of the food that you are eating. If you are used to eating carbohydrate-heavy meals, slowly change your diet to include more fruits and vegetables until your portions start to consist of mostly vegetables and whole foods. If you eat white bread or grain products, work on not eating them or even substituting them for healthier options like sprouted breads or wheat or brown carbohydrates. This incremental beginning can help you be more successful when you ramp up to more intense versions of intermittent fasting such as skipping days at a time.

Once you begin fasting, you can start journaling and keeping track of what you are eating. I like to use an old-fashioned pen and paper to track my daily meals in a food journal. However, one of the easiest ways to keep track of your calories and food choices is by using technology. Since our phones are already near us, you can easily use your phone as a resource to help you with your intermittent fasting journey. You can use your phone to choose an app that helps with your fasting. A couple of the most popular choices include Body Fasting app or Fitness Pal. Some apps have extra bonuses you can use, like hiring a personal health coach for extra support. As you keep track of your journey, do not forget to take note of your victories! Celebrate them. Perhaps you've been fasting three days in a row and are on track to fat perfectly for a week! Celebrate that! When you are tracking your food, take notes of certain trends. Are you meeting your calorie guidelines? Do you notice any trends about when you are mindlessly snacking or eating because you are stressed or because you didn't plan your meals well. Being able to track this information can help you create practices to help you combat your weaknesses.

On the other hand, if you end up going over on your calorie count one day, that's ok. The next day is a new day, and you should just get back on track and do not get too bogged down if you do not meet your goal. Your journal will also help you see if you are being serious or not.

You may trick other people, but you cannot fool yourself. Your journal will reflect if you need to give yourself a stern talking to or if you are being committed to being healthy or not. While what you eat is very important to maintaining your intermittent fasting lifestyle, it is not the only important thing. You should also make sure that you are getting enough sleep and exercising as well. If you like to bedazzle your personal items, now is the time to do it. Personalize your journal so that it's your own because it's going to be an important part of your intermittent fasting journey.

The longer you stay up, the more chances you have of eating more food. Sleeping helps with your fasting, and it also helps keep your cortisol levels low. Cortisol is a hormone that helps regulate your sleep. High levels of cortisol can potentially lead to insomnia. Intermittent fasting helps you sleep more peacefully, calmly and through the night. And by sleeping, it helps with your fasting a mutually beneficial relationship. When you add in exercise to the intermittent fasting equation, it only helps you have a better night's rest as well as compounding your intermittent fasting results.

Calculate Your Calories

One of the major tricks of being successful at fasting is to make sure that you have meals prepared so you will not be tempted to eat things that aren't good for you or overeat. In order to get those meals prepared ahead of time, you will want to have a pantry of your necessities in order to get those meals planned, but you have no idea how to begin. The first thing we will discuss is the approach to take. The first approach is easy. Since you already eat certain foods on a daily basis, find healthier recipes for the meals that you are already eating. The next way is to build your meals ahead of time. When planning a meal, you can try to have three different colors – a fruit, veggie, bean or a whole-wheat grain. You will also want to try to cook foods a healthy way like steaming, baking or roasting instead of frying and grilling. Cooking at home will definitely help you save more calories than eating out. (However, if you must eat out, look for the healthiest alternatives you can find.)

One way to prepare your meals ahead of time is to assemble the ingredients and freeze them. So when it is time to make your meal, you can thaw the ingredients and make them. Another way to prepare your meals ahead of time is to prepare your entire meal, like casseroles or easily freezable recipes, and then un-thaw them ahead of time and prepare them. As you start to fast more and more, you will discover what meals are your favorites and which meals are the easiest to prepare. To give you an idea of what types of healthy ingredients you can stock up on before you being meal planning follows.

- Proteins -Beans, quinoa, lean meats, nuts, peanut butter or your favorite type of nut butter
- Vegetables – Kale, spinach, lettuce, broccoli, mixed veggies, (The more vegetables you have, the merrier!)
- Fiber – Oatmeal, lettuce
- Fruit – Fresh, canned and frozen. Be careful of the sugar content in canned and frozen fruits to make sure unnecessary sugar is not being added.
- Healthy fats – Nuts, seeds, olive oil and coconut oil, oily fish like salmon and tuna
- Carbohydrates – brown rice, wheat breads, and sprouted breads
- Vitamins – Fish oil, Vitamin C, your favorite brand of all-purpose vitamins

You want to eat whole foods that contain lots of macronutrients. Macronutrients you want in your food include carbohydrates, fat, protein, minerals, vitamins, and water. I also want to make fiber an honorable mention. When you eat food with high levels of fiber, your digestive health improves. A simple rule of thumb is to keep your plate with as many varied colors as possible. Foods to consider eating are going to be lots of leafy vegetables like kale, swiss chard, greens, and lettuce; dark fruit like blackberries, raspberries, and strawberries, and drink lots of water even if you are already drinking lots of water. You can look into getting protein from non-meat sources such as nuts, quinoa or beans.

Do not forget to avoid worthless calories or foods that do not contain much nutrients that will keep you full, especially foods with lots of sugar. Sugar is everywhere! It is one of the most difficult things to cut out of your diet. However, if you want intermittent fasting to work, you will definitely want to be diligent against sugar. An ingredient to look for would be ingredients that end in 'ose' or anything that says 'high fructose corn syrup.' Easy ways to give up sugar is to gradually get rid of them by eliminating the most obvious culprits that have a high sugar count such as candy, soda (diet or otherwise), or juice. Also, giving up carbohydrates helps you rid yourself of the sugar. By eating whole foods with a dense nutrient count, it will help you avoid those cravings until you no longer even want sugar. While alcohol is not forbidden, it is one of those foods that take up calories without giving you many nutrients in return. Also, be mindful of those sneaky sugar calories in workout drinks or salty post-workout snacks that do not really help you enjoy the benefits of your workout! Additionally, when you go out to eat, try to have a peek at the menu in advance and try to pick out the options that fit into your calorie count.

Other quick notes to remember are:

- Snacks and drinks add extra calories to your meal so be mindful of what you are eating and drinking throughout the day. Are you eating and drinking because you are hungry or because you are bored?
- Make a grocery list and prep for the week. This will save you time and money!
- Have fun searching for recipes. To add some variety to your menu, try new ones! Being healthy is a positive so have fun

with it! Your meal planning is adjustable, so you do not have to feel boxed in.
- When you meal prep, do not feel like you have to do everything in one day. You can cut your vegetables one day and make your sauces on the next day. You can also, go ahead and prepare the ingredients, even the spices you are going to use beforehand so that the cooking will be seamless.

One way to amplify the benefits of fasting is if you pair your fasting with a vegan or vegetarian diet. Vegan diets consume no animal products such as eggs or honey. Vegetarians do not consume any meat, but they are allowed to eat eggs and products made by animals. Another popular diet to pair your intermittent fasting with is the ketogenic diet. Ketogenic diet is rich in proteins, fats and limits carbohydrates. This diet is great and trying to prevent seizures as well. Even if you do not want to partake in one of these diets, the intermittent lifestyle is still great for you. As long as you are staying within your caloric limit for the day and within your fasting window, you are ok. You can incorporate it into your lifestyle not matter if you cook at home or go out to eat.

If you want to go vegetarian or vegan, here a few tips that can help!

- For dairy milk, you can substitute any type of non-dairy milk like almond milk, soy milk or cashew milk. You can also make your own milk by soaking cashews in water overnight and then blending the cashews with water and adding extracts like vanilla or almond or whichever you prefer to give it extra flavor.
- For recipes that require yogurt, you can look into substituting a vegan alternative for yogurt.
- Butter, mayonnaise, cheese or cream cheese can be substituted for any vegan brand of the same product.
- There are many different ways to substitute eggs. You can use tofu instead of eggs if you are looking for a scrambled texture.

If you are using eggs to bind items in a recipe, you can use unsweetened applesauce, soft tofu, mashed bananas or the popular flax seed egg, which is just 1 tablespoon of ground flax seeds plus 3 tablespoons of water or another liquid and blend it all together. Then add the flax egg to the recipe.

- For meaty textures, you can try tofu. Use seitan or meatless meat. You can also use mushrooms or cauliflower, instead of meat, or even blended nuts to give it the same meaty texture.
- Instead of using honey, you can use agave, maple syrup, or any type of plant-based sweetener.
- There are also many different types of fish substitutions. You can search for your favorite vegan fish substitute to still enjoy fish recipes. Thankfully, there are a lot of vegan substitutes that are divine. When you incorporate them into your recipes, you won't be able to notice that you are having a vegetarian or vegan dish because it is as good as a dish with meat.

What Exercise Will Your Incorporate?

To determine what's the best exercise regimen for you to incorporate into your lifestyle, remember your why. Again, your goals will help you determine which exercise regime is best. No matter what exercise you do, it is recommended that you get at least 30 minutes of active exercise every day or 150 minutes a week to keep your heart healthy.

If you do not have money for a gym membership or personal trainer, one of the easiest ways to get a workout in, is to look for exercise routines online, especially on YouTube. There are a lot of free workouts on there. If you are sedentary most of the time and have a little extra money to spend, you can invest in a desk peddler or a standing desk so you can move while you are working. Another quick way to work out is to just do those basic old-fashioned exercises that you used to do in grade school, such as push-ups, sit-ups, jumping rope, and jumping jacks for thirty minutes. However, the key to this type of workout is to go as fast as you can and perform the exercises in sets. Perhaps you can do 3 sets of one exercise, rest, then do another three set of exercises and rest and keep going until you reach your 30 minutes. Exercise is something you definitely want to incorporate into your intermittent lifestyle if you want to maintain results and if you want to live healthily. Do not make excuses. Find a way to be active!

Of course, when you first start off fasting, you may take some time to get adjusted. To assist in meeting your weight loss goals, you may want to use a calorie counter. An easy way to track your calories throughout the day is to use a food journal. In the food journal, you will want to you notate the calories that you are consuming and the nutrient breakdown to make sure that you are meeting your goals. The more specific or strict you can determine how quickly you meet your health close. A food journal will also help you notice trends. What do you do before you eat bad foods usually? What are your cravings? Do they only happen on certain days or when you eat certain foods? Are you drinking enough water every day? These are all tips that can help you eat healthily and a great tool to pair with your fasting. This will be a valuable tool as you begin to get into the habit of intermittent fasting. If you need a little extra support, do not be afraid to look into health apps that offer health coaching. That may just be the extra boost you need. Health apps are truly popular and growing every day. You will be sure to find one that you need as long as you do a quick search on the App Store.

Do not be alarmed if you ever run into bumps. The key is to pick right back up where you left off. This chapter is a great one to come and visit for reference. We started off with three steps to help you get started intermittent fasting. You went over planning your meals, stocking your pantry, and making sure you are reaching your daily caloric limit, so you do not under eat or ovary. The chapter also the deeper into exercises you can incorporate to take your intermittent fasting to the next level. More importantly, this chapter offers some insight about what to do if you run into any plateaus or any issues while you are intermittent fasting. They are bound to happen, but the key is to keep going. Do not get discouraged. We all make mistakes. Have a short memory and pick up the next day if you are to ever fall short. A major tool for making your fasting journey work is the food journal that you should be keeping. Whether it is a hard copy or digital copy, a meal journal is key so you can know your personal trends and figure out the best practices that will work for you as you fast.

So what about hunger? You will get hungry at some point while fasting, but you will be able to overcome. Intermittent fasting takes advantage of our body's natural cycle of breaking down energy in our bodies. The way fasting works in the body is simple. Our bodies need energy to run. When we eat, we receive energy from the foods we eat like beans, vegetables, fruits, and carbohydrates to name a few. Our bodies then take sugar or glucose from the food and keep it stored in the muscles and liver. When our bodies need the energy, they release it into our bloodstream so our bodies can use it. Yet, when a person begins to fast, our bodies need to get the energy from a different source. After about eight hours of fasting, our livers use most of the glucose that is in our bodies. Our body then goes into gluconeogenesis, which indicates our body is about to enter fasting mode. When a person's body is in gluconeogenesis, this means that the calories that their body burns increases because if the body doesn't have any energy coming it, it makes its own glucose using your body fat. Once the body runs out of fat to use, it then begins to enter into starvation mode. Starving people are in a severe bodily mode in which their body is essentially eating itself to provide nutrients. This mode takes an extended amount of days and months to reach. It is not something that you can enter easily after a few hours of not eating. Intermittent fasting takes advantage of the gluconeogenesis mode that allows your body to burn more calories. This sweet spot of gluconeogenesis is where the leverage of intermittent fasting lies. You can safely fast for three days with water only by yourself. If you want to fast longer than three days with a water fast, be sure to touch base with your healthcare professional.

One of the major keys to surviving any fasting period is the importance of staying hydrated. It also helps you not enter starvation mode. Of course, you will want to drink water, but there are other liquids, you should be aware of. The key to drinking while fasting is to partake in drinks that have no calories. Here's a list of drinks you should consider drinking while fasting.

- Water- Water is one of the best liquids to consume while fasting. You can add a slice of lemon or infuse it with herbs, like basil, mint, or your favorite fruit. It is important to stay away from any sweeteners that can mess up your fast. This means you want to avoid sugary water enhancers like Crystal Light or any type of artificial flavoring to give the water more flavor. Enjoy the water as is and let it help you make it through the fast. To make your water fancier, you may even want to consider sparkling water. Mineral water is also great to drink during your fast.

- Broth - Any type of vegetable or bone -flavored broth can help you make it through a fast. If you can, you want to stay away from the store-bought broth that will have lots of extra sodium and flavors the best thing to do is to make your own broth. Broth is really helpful when you are fasting for longer than 24 hours.

- Tea - Any type of tea has proved to be extremely beneficial when you are fasting. Oolong, herbal, black, and green tea are all great to drink while you are fasting. Generally, tea improves your gut digestion, cellular detox, and balance of your probiotics. Be sure to watch the caffeine intake with the teas. It's good to go for caffeine-free options like ginger, chamomile, lemongrass, and hibiscus. You don't want to get addicted to caffeine or use it too much tea as an appetite suppressant while you are fasting. Peppermint tea helps get rid of your bloating and gas. Cinnamon chai tea is great to bust any sugar cravings you may have. Oolong and black tea lower your blood sugar. Lastly, green tea is great for an appetite suppressant.

- Apple cider vinegar -This is another type of liquid that can be very helpful during your fasting period as it helps improve your digestion and can help suppress your appetite.

- Coffee- Another great liquid to have during your fast is coffee. If you drink coffee, you want to make sure it does not cause an upset stomach or cause a racing heart. If drinking coffee does this to you, you may consider not drinking it. When drinking coffee in your fast, you also want to avoid using any artificial sweeteners, milk, or cream that will add extra calories. Avoid butter and coconut oil, too.
- If you want to flavor your coffee, consider adding spices like cinnamon, nutmeg or ginger for the bowl people.

- Smoothies- Smoothies are another great way to get the nutrition that you need. You can add vegetables to get the most out of your diet.

- Pureed Soups- These are great as well. You can even consider pureeing your favorite low-calorie meal if you want to stick to the liquid fast. This is another way you can get the nutrients that you need.

Now for the bad. Drinks you want to stay away from include sugary sodas, coconut water, juices, workout drinks like Gatorade or Powerade and definitely energy drinks. Almond milk is also a beverage you want to avoid while fasting. All these drinks have extra calories which will null-and-void your fast.

One more important thing to know about liquids is that it can help you beat symptoms of hunger while you are fasting. If you are having issues with dizziness or headaches, you will want to drink more water. Mineral water is also great for both of these issues. If you are having muscle cramps, you will want to drink water and soak in an Epsom salt bath to soak in. You may also consider taking a magnesium supplement. Lastly, if you are experiencing constipation, eat more fiber and drink more water during your eating period. You'll want to have more fruits, vegetables, and even chia seeds that have been soaked in a liquid like almond milk or even water if you're watching your calories. As long as you are consuming food during your eating windows, you will be ok. The next chapter will go into more detail about things to look out for when fasting.

The great thing about intermittent fasting is that it is pretty flexible. Therefore you are able to adjust your fasting days according to what's best for you and your body. If you need to go out to eat with friends or family during a time that is your normal fasting time, you can just adjust your window to make sure you meet the fasting requirements for the day, or you can make up the fasting time the next day. Another great thing about intermittent fasting is that you can drink water, black coffee or green or white tea during your fasting times to help you with your fasting periods. Weight loss is a welcome perk to intermittent fasting, but it is not the only perk. You may come to find that weight loss is just the cherry on top compared to other benefits of mental clarity and a lowered food bill.

For women, the best way to fast without throwing their hormones out of whack is to try to fast for 12 to 16 hours a day on two to three non-consecutive days. On the days that they fast, try to do light cardio or yoga. More intense workouts like strength or HIIT training can be done on the non-fasting days. Be sure to drink lots of liquids like tea, water, and coffee. If you are drinking tea and coffee, try not to put any sweetener or milk in it. You can also try to add a few amino acid supplements. If you feel comfortable, after 2 weeks, you can try to add another day of fasting. Not every woman is the same, and the results may vary per women. For women, it is important to go slowly and gradually to prevent adverse effects. Remember, you are not Superwoman or Superman, so take it slow to prevent hurting yourself and the people who care about you. Some people even like the form support groups of other minted fasters to encourage each other to keep going. This is especially helpful on the days that you want to work out. Exercising with others who understand what you're going through and who are going through the same thing with you can be empowering, encouraging, and helpful as you tried to stay the intermittent fasting path. Other still like to hire a trainer that is familiar with intermittent fasting to make sure if they are tapping into the best workout that can leverage the intermittent fasting lifestyle. Whether you want to work out by yourself or with others on YouTube or in person or with a trainer, it is advisable that you continue to work out and do not give up exercise just because you are intermittent fasting. Exercising is still part of having a healthy lifestyle.

When you are intermittent fasting, it is important to pay attention to your body! Keep a food journal if you can. (You can buy one online or use a digital one.) As a matter of fact, it is all advisable. (More will be given on this later in the book.) A person should always be aware of the effects are having on their body. You will know that your body is not responding positively to intermittent fasting. If at any time, you notice these things, you should stop.

- Insomnia – If you are consistently staying up all night, and just can't sleep, then you need to stop intermittent fasting, so

you look into the root cause of your insomnia further.
- Extreme hunger to the point that you can't do anything else unless you are thinking about food. – Intermittent fasting should be easy to do. Yes, at times, you will feel hunger. However, you should not be thinking about food so much that you are not able to function. There are a few tips you can use to alleviate your hunger pangs in Chapter 6 that can help you make it through your fasting windows. The truth of the matter once you get used to your fasting window, making it won't be an issue. The only concern you should have is if you can't make it through the intermittent fasting window and you cannot function AT ALL.
- Weight gain, specifically in your mid-area. – Unexpected weight gain, which is usually the opposite effect of intermittent fasting should be cause for concern. If at any point, you notice unexpected weight gain, you should definitely reach out to your doctor.
- Your period goes away or changes. – For women, this is extremely important. If you notice any abnormal changes to your period while fasting, you may need to stop. Long term issues with your period could cause fertility issues so if you notice anything, speak out. If you think your ovulation is at risk or you feel like you are running into fertility issues, please, please, please reach out to your doctor.
- You are especially stressed out. Intermittent fasting surprising helps people gain mental clarity. Many people have reported that they are sharper. However, if you feel utterly and completely overwhelmed, it is ok to stop fasting, especially if you have low energy and can't concentrate. If you feel that your performance has declined tremendously because of fasting, do not be afraid to stop.
- Skin and hair health – If you notice that your skin's color

looks off your hair seems thinner and brittle, this is a cause for concern. Any drastic changes with your hair and skin is an important indication that intermittent fasting isn't working.
- Decreased bone density and muscle tone decreases. – A change in your muscles or pain in your muscles can be a cause for concern. If you notice that your muscle tone has decreased or you feel pains doing your regular actions like walking the steps or getting in and out of cars, then you may want to reach out to your primary physician.
- You begin to have a change in digestion. – If at any point, you notice that you are having digestion issues that you were not having before, then intermittent fasting could be the cause. If there is extreme discomfort to where you cannot function, then reach out to your doctor. Some change in your digestion schedule is expected. However, if you notice something is way off, call the doctor.
- You are always cold. – Extreme coldness is another indication that you need to stop intermittent fasting. If you are colder than usual, and you have done everything you can to stay warm, but just can't stay warm. Then you need to reach out to your doctor.

The good news is that it is not all doom and gloom. However, there is a way to effectively practice intermittent fasting without falling into this vicious cycle, which is to gradually begin fasting. Do not begin all at once to prevent your body from going out of whack. More attention will be given to this in the next chapter. Ultimately, if you pay attention to your body, you will be able to tell if intermittent fasting is for you or not. Trust your body and listen carefully. It will let you know, so you do not have to be scared to try. Using the tips in this book will help you ease into the journey, so your body is not shell shocked.

When you fast, you need to also pay attention to the electrolytes that you are consuming. Electrolytes are the chemicals our bodies need to survive a fasted state. Electrolytes are already coming in our daily diet, but special attention should be given to them when you fast to make sure you are meeting your nutrient requirements in spite of fasting. Meeting the requirements are usually easy to do. As a matter of fact, most of us meet them every day without a hitch, but it is great to know what they are so you can be better prepared to handle intermittent fasting. After water, the most important ones are

- Calcium – This is found in leafy greens like collard greens, spinach, kale and sardines, and dairy. You will know you have a calcium deficiency if you have muscle spasms or bone issues.
- Potassium – This electrolyte can be found in bananas, plain yogurt, and potato skins. If you have mental confusion, weakness of the muscles or paralysis of the muscles, you may have a deficiency.
- Magnesium – Found in pumpkin seeds, spinach, and halibut, it is important to have this electrolyte. Confusion, nausea or muscle cramps are an indicator that you may be deficient in this electrolyte.
- Sodium – This electrolyte is in soup, salt, tomato juice, dill pickles, and tomato sauce. You know you may need this electrolyte if you have a loss of appetite or muscle cramps or dizziness.
- Chloride – If you have an irregular heartbeat or changes in your pH, you may be experiencing a deficiency in these electrolytes. It is found in veggies like tomatoes, olives, lettuce and table salt.

The most important electrolytes to have while fasting are magnesium, potassium, and sodium. You should have about a teaspoon of salt a day and mix it with water; 2000 milligrams of potassium and at least

300 to 450 milligrams of magnesium. When you are eating, as long as you are eating foods rich in these electrolytes it can sustain you during the fasted stated. Eating healthy during your eating windows is just as important as not eating during your fasting periods.

If you are still not sure if you can make it through the hunger pangs, here are some tips that can help. However, if you accept that hunger is a part of the fasting journey, you will have overcome one major hurdle. These tips can help you overcome and cope with hunger. They will be given as short-term strategies, long-term strategies, and a brief examination of what your craving and hunger can be telling you. By the time you finish reading, you'll be armed with all the necessary tools to bust hunger!

Short Term Strategies

When you are hungry, you want to eat immediately. You do not have time to think about long-term solutions to your hunger. You need something fast and efficient to help you cope so you can make it through your fasting window. The strategies in this section will help you do just that. These strategies are intended to help you with the here and now. Make a note of the ones you think that are specifically helpful. Choose 1 to 3 methods to lean on as you begin to help you cope with your hunger. You can play around with the different methods until you figure out which ones are the best for you.

- Eat a small snack. If you do eat a snack, go for a snack that under 50 calories and low-fat. If you must snack, make sure you include them in your meal planning efforts.
- Immediately distract yourself by playing a video game or another distraction to help you keep your mind off the hunger. If video games are not your thing, try to get distracted by pleasurable activities, especially ones that burn calories like taking a jog around the neighborhood or calling and speaking with a friend.

- Tap into the power of smell and smell something that smells like jasmine or vanilla. Both are shown to help crave sugar cravings.
- Take a nap. Sometimes hunger is an indication of being tired, not being hungry. The next time you are hungry, take a quick nap and see if the hunger resides once you wake up. Worst case scenario, the nap will serve as a distraction from your hunger and you will wake up not feeling hungry at all.
- When that hunger pang hits, floss and brush your teeth. You can even put a minty lip chap on with the hopes of the mint stopping you from getting too hungry. You can also pop a strong mint like an Altoid. The mint flavor should encourage you not to eat and mess up the freshness of your breath.
- Take a deep breath or do a few quick yoga poses to help clear your mind, and stop your cravings
- When your next craving hits, take the time to do for tea. Make a fancy tea time with a cup of hot tea. You can also do a nice cup of ginger tea as ginger has been shown to help stop cravings. Avoid sugary pastries and sweeteners during this tea time. You can also try fancy infused water, with mint, pomegranate, basil or cucumber or your favorite fruits instead. If tea or water isn't your thing, just make coffee instead. Remember, to limit the sweeteners and try to drink everything without creamer or sugar.
- Using acupuncture techniques is another way to try and curb your hunger. Tap your forehead for 30 seconds or try pinching your earlobes and nose.
- Another popular remedy to curbing your hunger is to chew gum, especially after lunchtime. Chewing gum can help you make it to your next eating window. Be sure to go for the sugarless variety. If you notice that you have any stomach issues after chewing gum for a long period of time, select a

different, hunger coping mechanism.
- Use your imagination and let yourself give in mentally. Imagine yourself eating whatever you want as a way to satisfy your hunger.
- Think about how eating your craving will affect you in the future. Will eating bring you closer or further away from your goals. Thinking of the long-term effects of not sticking to your fast may prevent you from eating during the fasted state.
- Just ignore the hunger pains. They typically last for 15 minutes. They come in bursts. If you can hold off for 15 minutes, you should be home free.
- Take a spoonful of apple cider vinegar after you eat or even before a meal. If you take it after you eat, the apple cider will help you make it through your fasted window. If you take the apple cider vinegar before you eat, it can help curb your appetite before you eat. If you take a spoonful while you are hungry, it can help you make it through your intermittent fasting window.
- Worst case scenario just give in and eat. Eat a very small portion, chew slowly and enjoy it. If you really give in, try to forgive yourself. We aren't always perfect, and sometimes we have to eat. However, try to go without eating for as long as you can before you give in. Try not to make it a habit.

Long Term Strategies

The strategies in this section aim to help you create habits that will help you long term on your intermittent fasting journey. Depending on your personality and your budget, these strategies can be easy or more difficult to implement. These strategies are ones that you should try once you have figured out that you are committed to being an intermittent faster. Even if you are not committed after you give it a test drive, some of these methods will still help you monitor your food intake.

Ideally, your goal should be to incorporate these tips and let them become a habit to help to make intermittent fasting for your easier.

- Try to coordinate your intermittent fasting with your schedule you are already following. Keep in mind that after about five hours, unless you are sleeping overnight, your blood sugar levels drop and you begin to crave food. If you can craft your fasting and eating windows with this concept in mind, it will be easier with you to deal with your hunger.
- Try to avoid purchasing high fructose corn syrup, because it is an additive. If you eat something with high fructose corn syrup in it, you will tend to want more of it. If you want some, it can cause you to want more. Other names high fructose syrup go by includes: fructose, maize syrup, glucose syrup, fructose or glucose syrup, tapioca syrup, fruit fructose, crystalline fructose or HFCS. Anytime you see one of these names your intermittent fasting antennae should be up and you should try and avoid that food.
- Next, try to avoid eating refined sugar which is often found in white sugar, white flour or white pasta. Try to replace it with natural sweeteners, nut flours, or whole grain pasta or forgo these ingredients all together.
- Purchase blue plates for your home. Blue plates are shown to help prevent cravings. This may be a little pricey so do not be afraid to check second-hand stores for this item. Also, try using smaller plates that will help limit your portions sizes. You can also use bigger forks which help you feel fuller faster.
- Try to get more sleep. If we do not get enough sleep, that's when you can begin trying to compensate with unhealthy eating choices. Sleeping is so important to a healthy lifestyle. This is one area where you do not want to skimp on. Give yourself seven to eight hours a night and watch the difference

it will have in your life. Your mood will improve, your weight will improve, and your productivity will improve. Sleeping is underrated. Give it a try and watch how it affects your life.

- Create a list of items to do that calms you, makes you happy or that you enjoy. Try to let them be things that do not involve eating. Try to create 25 things and pick one the next time you are hungry pick one from the list.
- Are you an emotional eater? If so, try to get to the root cause of why you are eating when you are emotional. Remember that journal you were supposed to keep from earlier? Be sure to note any trends of when you are eating if you are bored, stressed, sad, or mad, then adjust your behavior accordingly. Be mindful of what you are eating so you do not eat because you are bored or stressed.
- Just like hunting for high fructose syrup or refined sugars, get into the habit of reading food labels. You'll want to pay special attention to the serving size. This will help you not if you are overeating or not. Also, saturated fats and sodium are other categories that you want to pay attention to and choose foods that are high in fiber. When you add more fiber to your meal, it helps you make it through your fasting periods easier. You'll also want to pay special attention to the vitamins and minerals in the food to make sure it is full of good food for you.
- Make the lights brighter when you eat your meals. This is an interesting tip and may be on the pricey side if you need to buy a few new or brighter bulbs. Bright lights raise the awareness of what you are eating; whereas, dim lights tend to lower your inhibitions. This means when the lights are low, you tend to overeat. Keep those lights bright, so you do not overeat and effectively ruin your intermittent fasting eating window.

- Another quick way to help you watch what you eat and prevent you from overeating during your window is to have a soup or salad as an appetizer first. You can also have a cup of water first. This tip can fill you up with good nutrients and help you not to overeat.
- Although it sounds counterintuitive, you will want to eat the same foods every day. This helps your body to adjust easier and helps make meal planning easier to make sure you are getting the proper nutrients and calories that you need. If you are a person, who believes that spice is the variety of life. Do not be afraid to try new things after at least eating a set schedule for a few days to see how your body reacts. The best to back your diet is with foods that are bulky but low in calories like whole grains, beans, fruits, and vegetables.

Whether you are interested in adding short-term or long-term strategies to your life, both of these categories can help you make it when you feel like your stomach is going to fall through your back. Again, pick one to two strategies to start with, and note them in your food journal. You will be able to track and see which methods work the best for you and which ones are keepers and which ones you need to replace. The next section will deal with a different aspect of your hunger. It will focus on your cravings and how to tell if your cravings are telling you something or not. What our cravings tell us can be especially helpful to our meal planning and overall health.

What your cravings are telling you!

We all get hungry, but some of us never pay attention to what we are craving for at the moment. In order to survive, our bodies want certain nutrients, vitamins, and minerals to sustain us. Sometimes, we just want good ol' water. The following section details what our cravings could be telling us. When you are writing in your food journal, pay special attention to what you are craving and what days. Noting the time and if you are craving these foods after any certain activities will also provide insight into what you are craving.

Keeping careful track of your cravings can help you figure out what you are craving and, in some cases, why. It will help you take your combatting hunger to another level. By focusing on what your hunger is telling you, you are making sure you are meeting your dietary needs as well as possibly catching any disturbing signals that your body may be telling you. Sometimes our bodies give similar signals for certain cravings, but the best thing to do if you are not sure what to do is to drink water. It typically helps with cravings and satiates hunger. Do not underestimate the power of paying attention to what your body is telling you. Listen and watch your body reward you for it.

If you are craving salty foods...

This is a good indicator that you need to drink more water. Our body responds to being dehydrated by craving salty foods. This is a common craving people have. If you have it, let an 8-ounce cup of water sooth it. Along with water, increase your intake of calcium, magnesium, and zinc. Make sure that you are not experiencing exhaustion, extreme weight loss or a change in the color of your skin. This could point to a larger healthy issue if you are craving salt all the time. To encourage you to drink more water, you can purchase a cool water bottle or personalized one that you already have to your liking. This will give a special touch to your water drinking. If you are a person who despises water, see if you can start with sugarless sparkling water or invest in sparkling water machine to make your own sparkling water at home. You can also consider infusing the water with different fruits to give it a taste. There are no ways around not drinking water. You just have to find a way to cope with drinking it that is to your liking.

If you are craving sweet food...

Just like salty foods, a sugar craving is a good indicator that you need to drink more water. This craving is also related to your caffeine intake and your sleeping schedule. A sugar craving can also be your body's way to stay energized. So if you down lots of caffeine and barely are getting any sweets, try to get some sleep and lay off the caffeine as well. Another way to help ease this craving is to incorporate more naturally sweet fruits and vegetables into your diet, like carrots, sweet potatoes, beets, apples or vegetables into your diet. Instead of sugar, you can try natural sweeteners such as agave or maple syrup instead of sugary snacks and drinks. Honey is touted as helping you feel full longer so do not overlook this favorite sweetener or many. If you are always craving something sweet, try something sour to kill the craving. Sour foods also help improve your digestive system. Lastly, incorporating more protein in your diet can also help you overcome sugary diet as your body will be sustained and you do not have to rely on sugar to pick your body up.

If you are craving chocolate, cheese, and dairy products...

If you are craving chocolate or cheese, you may need to pick up your mood. Chocolate and cheese are known as comfort foods and rightfully so since they release feel-good chemicals to improve your mood. If you notice that you are having these types of cravings, look for ways to boost your mood like taking a quick jog or doing a few quick stretches at your desk. If you are still struggling with chocolate and dairy cravings after trying to improve, you can consider looking into vegan options or eliminating it from your diet altogether. Ridding themselves of dairy has helped a lot of people with their health journey, and if you do that on your intermittent fasting path, you may be surprised at the results.

If you are craving ice or red meat...

This could point to an iron deficiency. If you have low iron, increase your protein intake or even eat more red meat. If you are vegan or vegetarian, see about increasing your intake with beats of plant-based sources or protein. Make sure this craving is not coupled with any drastic skin or hair changes, as well. Iron is an important aspect of a healthy lifestyle, so don't overlook this craving if you have it.

If you are craving soda...

Craving a carbonated, sugary soda suggests that you may have a calcium deficiency. Increase your calcium intake to help with this craving. You can find calcium in leafy green vegetables if you are vegan and other plant-based sources so do not feel that you only can find calcium in dairy. If you are craving the carbonation so you can burp, try sparkling water or club soda with fruit infused in it to see if it will give you that same field. Sparkling water is a much healthier option than soda, and it gives you some of the same joys of burping that soda does.

If you are craving French fries and potato chips...

A craving such as this means that you need to eat more healthy fats found in oily fish like salmon, sardines or nut. If this is a persistent craving, you should also consider adding more fiber, magnesium and chromium food that is found in foods like chard, celery, spinach, apricots, apples, and bananas. If you just can't seem to rid yourself of the potato chip or French fry craving, create your own healthier options from sweet potatoes or white potatoes. You can also thinly sliced vegetables and create your own crunchy vegetables by roasting them with a little extra virgin olive oil in the stove. These are healthier alternatives, and you may become addicted to them just like you are to French fries and chips, which would not be a bad problem to have.

Any other craving no matter how weird or bizarre...

Drink more water to try to help the craving. Also, note if you can tell any weird other things happening with your body such as extreme weight loss or weird mood swings or any other dramatic changes. Some food cravings can point to pregnancy if you are a woman or other health issues for men and women. Always err on the side of caution. If you feel like something weird is going on, trust your instincts. Health Care Providers are there for a reason. Don't be afraid to reach out to them.

If you are eating a well-balanced diet, then your craving issues should be easier to manage and control. Not just a well-balanced diet, but drinking a lot of water is helpful, too. The next section will focus on more tips to help you get through your non-eating periods and answers any questions you may have.

Chapter 4: Fasting Tips and FAQs

When you begin fasting, it is important to make notes in your food journal. It will give you insight on how you can manage your fasts better and longer. So when you get super-duper hungry, and you do not know how to stop your hunger, you'll look at your food journal. Your food journal notes will help you see what cravings you are normally having? Are you eating whole foods and foods with lots of fiber? Do you notice any other trends or have tried any other recipes to help with your hunger? If so, some other ways to curb your hunger pangs are:

- Distract yourself! Sometimes you have to focus on something else so you will not focus on the hunger.
- Learning how to deal with your hunger pangs. Initially, you are going to feel hungry. If you can train your mind that it will last only a little while, and they typically do, you will be able to pick right back up and make it to your next meal.
- Consider avoiding snacks. There have been people to say that snacking throughout the day helps lose weight. The truth is that the total number of calories determine whether if you lose weight. So if you are a snacker and you need them to function, continue to do so as long as the snack does not interfere with your daily calorie count. However, try to take them out and just eat the main meals during your eating period to see if you notice a difference or not.

- When you eat, make sure you are chewing at least 30 times before you swallow. This makes sure that you are properly digesting your food, enjoying the flavors and slowing down your meal to make sure you are not overeating.
- Also stopped eating a little bit before you feel full and drink water. This is another good tip to help you prevent overeating.

- Next, try not to sleep after you eat. This won't help you as you try to become more efficient with fasting. It will actually hinder your progress.
- Drink lots of water and do not forget to take your vitamins. Water is an important way to intermittent fast successfully.

Fasting is indeed a lifestyle, and there are a few mistakes you want to be aware of once you begin. Knowing what they are beforehand will hopefully help you not to have to struggle with them at all. Even if you run into any bumps in the road, remember to get right back up and to keep going. You are not expected to be perfect the first time you try your hand at. With careful planning and perseverance, you will be intermittent fasting like a pro in no time. These are some of the top mistakes that people make while they are intermittent fasting. Take notes and try to avoid them if you can.

1. Over-eating and Binge Eating – Avoiding overeating and binge eating during your time to eat is important. When it is time to eat, eat a regular sized portion and do not try to compensate for your fasting period. This overcompensation prevents you from taking advantage of your intermittent fasting period.
2. Not Eating Enough - When you eat, do not feel like you can't eat. Take advantage of your eating period, but do not gorge yourself. Make sure you are eating healthy food and not junk. If you make sure your food is full of macronutrients, you will be able to make it through your fasted states easier.
3. Not Drinking Enough Water – Water is the life force of us all and staying hydrated is a major key to making the intermittent lifestyle work for you. Staying hydrated prevents cravings and helps you make it through the fasting period. Do not neglect this important step.
4. Not Choosing the Right Method – Intermittent fasting

should be easy. If it feels like you have to work too much or it is not flowing with your lifestyle, do not be afraid to try a new method. There is not a hard and fast rule about which method is the best. Whichever method you choose should fit into your lifestyle. Remember, this is a lifestyle change and not a diet. You can take the time to figure out which method works the best for you.

5. Obsessing Too Much - If you weigh yourself obsessively or worrying about if you are doing intermittent fasting, take a deep breath and relax. Results can take time. You shouldn't expect drastic change overnight. Just relax and take your time. Before you know it, you will see the benefits that are extremely helpful.

6. Giving Up Too Soon – Do not join the many other people who threw in the towel too soon on intermittent fasting. Give yourself about two weeks to measure the results and see if it is working or not. Do not just give up after a day or two. This method is proven throughout time to work. This tricky part is finding which method works out the best for you. Keep playing around with it and do not give up too soon. However, remember if at any point, you begin to experience drastic results, it may be time to throw in the towel.

Ultimately, if you are food journaling, you will be able to pick up on some of these mistakes that you make. Any time you noticed a mistake, try to find a way to correct it with a better practice. Be gentle and kind to yourself and keep going. You will soon realize that intermittent fasting and fasting is not that bad.

Frequently Asked Questions

At this point, I am sure that you have a lot of questions that you need to be answered about fasting and myths that need to be busted. For those who are on the fence or those who are excited to begin, this section will be especially helpful. It will go over some common myths that may give you pause before beginning as well as alleviate some of the fears you may have. Hopefully, by the time you finish reading, you will be ready to get started fasting!

<u>Will I get the keto flu?</u>

The keto occurs as your body adjusts to the keto diet. Symptoms include increased hunger, nausea, and decreased energy. To help aid your transition to a keto diet, you will want to go slowly when eliminating carbs. After a few days, your body should adjust. If you have extreme side effects, be sure to reach out to your healthcare provider.

<u>If I'm doing the keto diet, aren't all carbs bad?</u>

All carbohydrates are not bad, but since the keto diet is low-carb, you will want to limit your carbohydrates intake. The keto diet is a low-carb diet, not a no-carb diet, so you will need to eat carbohydrates at some point, but you just make smart decisions when eating carbohydrates if you are on the keto diet.

<u>Isn't every carbohydrate sugar?</u>

A potato and a candy bar are not the same thing. It is important to understand that sugar, or sucrose, is the unhealthy type of sugar. Grains and potatoes and other healthy starches turn into glucose which is a form of sugar that can raise blood sugar in diabetic patients. The main difference is that sucrose is not a healthy type of sugar like glucose. No matter if you are eating sucrose or glucose, the key is moderation.

<u>Aren't potatoes, carrots, and fruit unhealthy because of carbohydrates?</u>

If you are doing the keto diet, yes, you will want to limit these types of foods, but this does not mean that they are inherently unhealthy. These foods are great to eat, and if you are doing the keto diet, you will want to watch how you eat them. Knowing why you're doing the keto and counting your calories is very important when you are doing the keto diet.

<u>The keto diet is the best diet for everyone, right?</u>

The keto diet is not necessarily the best diet for everyone. You will need to check with your healthcare provider first to make sure that it is the best diet for you. The keto diet has many health benefits, so it is important to know why you are doing it so it can fit your body's type and lifestyle.

<u>How do I get over the mental block of not eating?</u>

If you do not eat, you feel like you are starving. Ever had this feeling? No worries, you are not alone. This is a common feeling to have. Sometimes when we get that feeling, it doesn't mean that we're always hungry. It can mean that you are thirsty instead. If you are having trouble overcoming this barrier, think about what you can do when you do get this feeling. What's your plan of action going to be? How about drinking a glass of water, listening to your favorite song or doing your favorite activity until the feeling passes? I'll be honest. The mental block of not being able to eat is one of the most difficult barriers overcome when doing intermittent fasting, but it is not difficult to overcome once you get in the habit of doing it. Once you make it through, you will realize that it will get easier and easier until your body gets used to the fasting period and your eating period.

There are a lot of questions that people have about intermittent fasting and the validity of how it can help improve your overall health. This chapter addresses some of the most common misconceptions and frequently asked questions one may have about intermittent fasting. Hopefully, after reading this chapter, if you are on the fence, you will be convinced about the positives about intermittent fasting.

<u>What's the best diet to couple intermittent fasting with?</u>

Great question. There is not an 'official' one. It depends on your goals. If you want to lose more weight, popular diets to pair with intermittent fasting are vegan, vegetarian or keto diets. More important than diet is the importance of eating a well-balanced diet not matter which dietary option you decide upon and stay within our caloric limits.

<u>Can I use the ketogenic diet to intermittent fast if I am diabetic?</u>

Some people have coupled intermittent fasting with a keto diet with some success. However, there are still studies being done to determine if this is the best way to do intermittent fasting with diabetes. There are some benefits to intermittent fasting with diabetes like regulation of your insulin and glycogen levels. However, the most important step is to talk with your healthcare provider before deciding to take this journey.

<u>Is it safe?</u>

Yes. For healthy adults, intermittent fasting should not be an issue. You may even realize that there are many more benefits to intermittent fasting than you thought. However, for those who are elderly, pregnant, breastfeeding or taking medication, check with your healthcare provider first.

<u>How much can I train on an empty stomach?</u>

The most difficult part of training while intermittent fasting is to let your body get used to it. When your body gets used to working out while fasting, you will realize that you may get extra strength and energy to do your workout. When you train while you fast, your workout can be more efficient and help you burn more calories or build more muscle. So if you can handle training on an empty stomach go for it. Ultimately, it is up to you and your exercise goals to decide what you can handle.

Many people decide to train during their eating window so they can eat a pre and post workout meal. If you are trying to lose weight, foregoing your pre-workout meal will help you lose more weight. Just remember that after your work out, try to eat protein and fiber to rebuild your body from the workout. Others also find that eating more carbohydrates on the days that they work out, helps them with the workouts.

<u>Can I just eat fruits as a main meal?</u>

It is best to eat a balanced diet. Too much fruit could give you too much sugar and give you unwanted weight gain if you do it too often. If you prefer fruits, try to disguise your greens by adding your greens with your fruits in a juice blend or smoothie.

<u>What are the side effects?</u>

You may experience headaches, diarrhea, cramps, and discomfort. You may also experience insomnia, lower back pain, and hair loss. But if you experience these, reach out to your health care provider since these are extreme side effects. The most common side effects are hunger pangs, headaches, and discomfort. You should not feel totally lethargic or as if you cannot function by missing a meal or two a day. If you try intermittent fasting and you have just horrible side effects, it may not be for you, and that is okay.

<u>How do I help with my hunger pangs?</u>

One way to help with your hunger is to drink lots of liquid especially water. You can drink a big glass of water when you wake up or anytime you experience hunger pangs. What's more, you can put Himalayan salt in your water to give it an extra boost. You can also drink tea, amino acids, and coffee as much as you'd like, too. Just watch the extras like milk, cream, and sugar.

<u>How can I tell if intermittent fasting or fasting is working?</u>

One way to tell if it is working or not is to look at your body. Are you losing weight? How do you feel? Do you feel like you are sleeping better? Do you have a clearer mind or energy boost? Do you feel happiness generally? These are factors to look at when deciding if it is the right lifestyle for you or not. It is also important to note which method of intermittent fasting works best for you.

<u>Why should I skip breakfast? Is not breakfast the most important meal of the day?</u>

Wonderful question. The word breakfast means to break the fast. This idea that breakfast is the most important meal of the day is from an outdated diet concept. The typical American diet consists of sugary breakfast options like waffles, pancakes, pastries, etc. If you are not going to eat a healthy breakfast, why eat it anyway? Making sure you have enough calories throughout the day is more important than when you eat it. So if you eat your first meal at lunch, then your 'breakfast' would be your 'lunch.' Eating breakfast or not is totally up to your body and whether you and your body can handle it or not. The great thing is if you need breakfast to function, just make it a part of your eating window and make sure you are eating a healthy option for breakfast. Most people tend to skip breakfast, so that's why skipping breakfast is not a major issue for most people. However, listen to your body and do what's best for your body's natural cycle.

Is not it healthier to eat more meals throughout the day?

This is a great question, too. The nutrients in your food and the number of calories you are eating is more important than when you eat it. If your body responds to smaller meals through the day, go ahead. If your body responds more to larger meals, feel free to do so. It is more important to make sure that you are not overeating your daily caloric limit than when you eat those meals.

If you partake in intermittent fasting, will you develop an eating disorder?

Intermittent fasting is not about developing an extreme eating pattern. It is a controlled pattern of eating during a certain time and not eating during another time. It is best matched up to your natural eating habits. The foods you eat are nutrient dense, so they are oftentimes healthier eating options that the foods you already partake in eating. Most people who do intermittent fasting do not develop an eating disorder. They actually become healthier from this lifestyle. However, if you have a history of eating disorder or are concerned that you may develop one by beginning, consult your healthcare professional before beginning.

Does intermittent fasting or fasting cause you to overeat?

Interesting, when you begin intermittent fasting, the exact opposite tends to happen. Unless you are purposefully overeating, you will find that your appetite tends to change and you start to crave smaller portions. Remember, American portions are many times larger than what normal portions are across the world so the smaller portions would be considered normal portions worldwide.

<u>Will I start to starve?</u>

Gandhi was able to go on a hunger strike, only drinking water, and did not die. A few extended hours between meals is not going to cause you to starve or die. Our bodies normally have about a month's worth of stored fat available to us every day. So you will have a constant energy supply even if you intermittently fast.

<u>Will I gain weight if I eat later in the day or late at night?</u>

The best thing about intermittent fasting is that it fits into your lifestyle. You can choose to decide when to eat your meals. Of course, if you are eating lots of carbohydrates only, overeating and not eating vegetables or fruit with a late eating window, you may gain weight. The key is moderation and balance. If you are eating a normal portion at night, you should not see weight gain. Again, it depends on your body. Keep notes in your food journal to see how your body reacts to eating at a later window. If you are operating at a calorie deficit, you should be fine. The most important thing is not to overeat to avoid giving yourself a stomach ache and extra calories.

<u>Will I lose a lot of muscle when I intermittent fast or fast?</u>

When you eat, your body releases the nutrients you need steadily over time. Until you need to replenish nutrients from your next meal. Many people assume that fasting immediately causes muscle loss which is not the case at all. When you fast, remember you are still using the nutrients from your previous meal even if it was 16 to 20 hours ago. So realistically you will not lose muscle weight just by fasting in a certain window.

As you continue to learn about intermittent fasting, you will be surprised that it is actually quite healthy and has lots of benefits. Most of the misconceptions about intermittent fasting are resolved once you start practicing and see how the positive effect it has on your body.

Plateauing

After you start fasting, you may run into a few issues. You have lost a couple of pounds, but now you are not sure how to lose more. You've seemed to flatline. What do you do next? This section is all about how to maintain the weight you have lost and how to overcome any ruts you may run into.

First things first. Here are a few questions to ask yourself about how to maintain your weight. When you initially start intermittent fasting, you may see huge results, but if at any time you begin to eat more and not exercise portion control, there is the chance you may gain that weight back. However, there are some ways to try and monitor your weight so you can stay on the straight-and-narrow intermittent path.

- When you look in your food journal or your calorie are you still eating the same number of calories? Has that number changed at all? If so, why? And how can you fix it? What other weird trends do you notice? For example, on days that you are busy, you notice that you always break your fast? How can you fix some of the challenges on the trends that you see?
- Are you drinking enough water? Sometimes you are not hungry; you are dehydrated and drinking more water can prevent you from eating worthless calories.
- Are you binging during your meals when you can eat or are you eating normal potions? It is expected that you may gain some weight back if you are eating double portions to compensate for when you are not eating. The idea is to keep the same amount of food that you are eating so your body can

reap the benefits of a true fasting period.
- Additionally, what types of foods are you eating? Has the method you have chosen fit easily into your current lifestyle or are you having a difficult time fasting with the current method you've chosen. Are you only eating carbohydrates like bread and pasta with limited fruits and vegetables? If you must have some of your favorite unhealthy foods, see if you can find a vegetarian or vegan or a healthier version of that recipe.
- Have you tried a different fasting window? Sometimes a different window can help you get better results. You can play around with different fasting windows until you find the one that works the best for you.
- How is your sugar intake? Are you still eating sugar in high amounts or even eating foods that have those sneaky sugar calories hidden inside them? A review of the ingredients in the foods that you eat can help you find the culprit.
- Are there any days where you are feeling dizzy, nauseated, fatigued or having difficulty concentrating? What are the foods that you are eating when you notice these symptoms? This will help you figure out if the food you are eating is agreeable or if you need to eat more or less of certain foods.
- Are your meals well-balanced? Do you see a lot of different colors from different food groups on your plate when you eat or only one type of color?
- How fast did you transition to intermittent fasting? Are you getting enough calories for your energy needs? If you are drastically below the recommended count for women or men, you may need to eat more.
- Are you eating enough when you work out? Are you carb cycling which means you eat a slightly bigger portion on the days you workout to help you have a great workout versus the

days when you do not work out.
- Are you having trouble binging on sugar or having a difficult time breaking bad habits? If so, perhaps you can allow yourself at least 3 cheat meals a month to satisfy those cravings.
- What type of exercises are you doing? Are the exercises complementary to weight or muscle gain? If the exercises you are doing are helping you gain muscle, like lifting weights, you may not be losing weight, but you are gaining muscle which can help you lose weight in the long term. More cardio based exercises can help you burn more calories and potentially lose more weight. Be sure to make sure your exercise regimen is helping you reach your goals.

Mind you, if you were to stop at all, you might gain some of the weight that you've lost. So keep going! Do not give up. The race is not to the swift but to those who endure, be mindful that you may not see changes because you are with your body all the time. However, if you ask someone else, they may be able to point out changes that you are not aware of so do not be afraid to ask for a second opinion. Additionally, weight loss may not be the first benefits you see. Note your mood and your focus and your energy levels to see if intermittent fasting has made an impact on your life in other ways besides wait. Trust me; people will know and talk about it if they notice a difference. If they don't, that's okay too. Just ask for their honest opinion and see what they have to say if you need some validation. Just make sure the person that you're asking if someone that you trust and who has your best interest in mind.

Remember, if you do not see your expectations being met as quickly as you expect, it is okay to make a few changes to see if you can reach your goals. After tweaking a few things while you fast, and you still aren't meeting your expectations it may be time to get more realistic ones. Nevertheless, keep working with your intermittent fasting windows, your meal, and portion choices as well as your exercise routines until you get the results that you want. Mistakes and mishaps are inevitable, but it is important to keep a good sense of humor and a sense of determination so you can make it through. Hopefully, this chapter has put to rest any fear that you may have about intermittent fasting and assured you of the benefits that it has. Even if you do not decide to stick with intermittent fasting long-term, at least giving it a try will open your eyes to a new method of living and your body will thank you. Hopefully, you are convinced about all the benefits of intermittent fasting and fasting! The last chapter will give you a few recipes you can use to start your intermittent and fasting journey.

Chapter 5: Fasting Recipes

If you are not sure what to eat on the keto diet when you are intermittent fasting, this chapter is a great start. It gives you simple, quick recipes that you can use on your intermittent fasting journey. There are five recipes given for breakfast, lunch, dinner, and snacks. Enjoy!

Breakfast

Baked Eggs

This recipe takes about 10 minutes to prepare, 10 minutes to cook, and it makes 4 servings.

The serving size is two eggs, and it contains:

- 400 milligrams Cholesterol
- 13 grams Protein
- 204 milligrams Sodium
- 1 gram Sugar
- 1 gram Carbohydrates
- 9 Saturated fats
- 19 grams Total fat

What to Use

- Salt and Pepper (to taste)
- Unsalted butter (2 tbsp)
- Heavy cream (2 tbsp)
- Large eggs (8)
- Grated vegan cheese (1 tbsp)
- Fresh parsley (1 tbsp)
- Fresh rosemary (0.5 tsp)
- Fresh thyme (0.5 tsp)
- Fresh garlic (0.25 tsp)

What to Do

- Pre-heat your oven broiler for 5 minutes and place the oven rack about 6 inches below the heat.
- Combined all your herbs and cheese in a separate bowl and set it aside. Crack two eggs in four individual small bowls without breaking the yolk. You will not be baking them in this dish.
- Put 4 individual baking ramekins on a baking sheet. Put a 0.5 tbsp of cream and 0.5 tbsp of butter in each dish and place under the broiler for about 3 minutes until it's hot and bubbling. Take it out the oven and quickly, but very slowly, pour two eggs into each ramekin. Then sprinkle the herb mixture in each ramekin and add the salt and pepper. Put the dishes under the broiler for five to six minutes until the egg whites are almost cooked. Remember the eggs will cook when you take them out the oven.

Breakfast Salad

This recipe takes 5 minutes to prepare, 15 minutes to cook, and it makes 1 serving.

A serving contains:

- 17 grams Protein
- 3 grams Sugar
- 7 grams Fiber
- 13 grams Carbohydrates
- 29 grams Total fat

What to Use

- Salt (to taste)
- Avocado (0.3 of the avocado and make it sliced)
- Roasted cauliflower (0.5 c)
- Baby greens of kale, spinach or your favorite (2-3 c)
- Chopped red onion (0.25 c)
- Eggs 92-3)
- Olive Oil (2 tsp)

What to Do

- Sauté the onion until soft in the olive oil.
- Then add in the roasted cauliflower and green. Sprinkle with a salt.
- Then make the two eggs how you like it and put it on top of the salad.

Breakfast Patties

This recipe takes 30 minutes to prepare, and it makes 16 patties. A serving it 1 patty, and it contains:

- 10 grams Protein
- 275 milligrams Sodium
- 5 grams Total fat

What to Use
Cayenne Pepper (0.5 tsp)
Ground ginger (0.5 tsp)
Pepper (1 tsp)
Dried Sage leaves (1 tsp)
Salt (1.5 tsp)
Lean ground turkey (2 lbs)
What to Do

- Combine all the ingredients in a bowl. Then shape into the patties into 16 2.5 inches separate patties.
- In a large skillet cook about 4-5 minutes on each side until there is no pink left.

Avocado Zucchini

This recipe takes 5 minutes to make and makes 1 serving.
A serving contains:

- 14 grams Protein
- 3 grams Sugar
- 17 grams Fiber
- 43 grams Carbohydrates
- 977 milligrams Potassium
- 162 milligrams Sodium
- 6 grams MSG
- 5 grams Polyunsaturated fat
- 4 grams Saturated fat
- 24 grams Total Fat

What to Use

- Zucchini (cut and halved)
- Hemp hearts (1 tablespoon)
- Radishes (2 thinly sliced)
- Avocado (1 pitted and peeled)

What to Do

- Mash the avocado until it forms a past and spread half of it on one slice of zucchini.
- You can top with radishes and garnish with salt and pepper if desired.

Simple Chia Pudding

This recipe takes about 6 hours and 5 minutes to prepare and makes 4 servings.

The serving size is 0.5 g. It contains:

- 6.9 grams Protein
- 3 grams Sugar
- 9.5 grams Fiber
- 16.3 grams Carbohydrates
- 23 milligrams Sodium
- 4.3 grams Saturated fats
- 10.3 grams Fat

What to Use

- Extract (Vanilla) (1 teaspoon)
- Agave (1-2 tablespoons)
- Dairy-free milk (1.5 cups)
- Seeds - Chia (0.5 c)

What to Do

1. First, combine the maple syrup, vanilla extract, chia seeds, and dairy-free milk in a bowl. Then whisk the ingredients very well to mix them all together.

2. Refrigerate the ingredients overnight or for at least 6 hours in the bowl (preferably overnight), so the chia pudding is thick and creamy. If the chia pudding is not thick and creamy, you can add more chia seeds. Then, put it back into the refrigerator and keep it in there for about another hour or so until the pudding is firm. You can garnish it with fruit or almonds or nuts of your choice.

Lunch

Cauliflower Nachos with Turkey Meat

This recipe takes preparation time of 15 minutes, cooking time of 25 minutes, and creates 4 portions.

A serving contains:

- 27 g Protein
- 29 g Fat Total
- 14 g Carbohydrates
- 6 g Fiber
- 5 g Sugar

What to Use

- Fresh Cilantro (2 tbsp)
- Avocado (0.5 medium avocados)
- Red onion (sliced 0.3 cup)
- Tomatoes (diced 0.75 cup)
- Cheddar cheese (1 cup shredded)
- Turkey sausage (1 pound)
- Taco seasoning (1 tsp)
- Avocado oil (0.25 cup)
- Cauliflower (1 large head)
- Salsa (optional)
- Guacamole (optional)

What to Do

1. Start your oven up to 425 degrees. Put grease on your baking sheet and oil it well. Cut the cauliflower into florets and slice them as thinly as possible to make chips. Toss the cauliflower chips with the taco seasoning and avocado oil.

2. Roast them for about 20 minutes on the sheet as a single layer until browned and crispy on the edges.

3. While the cauliflower is roasting, go ahead and cook the turkey sausage for about 10-12 minutes until you do not see any pink.

4. When the cauliflower is finished roasting, flip them over and place the cooked meat over the top of it.

5. Add cheese, red onion, and tomatoes. Then let it in the heat till the cheese melts nicely.

6. You can garnish it with cilantro and avocado. You can add your favorite salsa and guacamole mix or chop a few tomatoes and avocado to make a tomato and avocado salad.

Skirt Steak with Red Pepper

This recipe takes 1 hour and 10 minutes to prepare, and it makes 4 servings.

A serving contains:

- 25 grams Protein
- 8 grams Sugar
- 3 grams Fiber
- 19 grams Carbohydrates
- 676 milligrams Sodium
- 10.4 grams MSG
- 1.5 grams Polysaturated Fat
- 5.2 grams Saturated Fat
- 18.2 grams Total fat

What to Use

- Salt and Pepper (to taste)
- Olive oil (2 tbsp)
- Water (1 c)
- Red bell peppers (divided into two)
- Skirt steak (1 lb)
- Green onions (0.75 c chopped and divided)
- Fish sauce (3 tbsp)

What to Do

- To begin this recipe, start off making the marinade. Mix about 0.3 cups of the onion and fish sauce in a shallow bowl. Coat the steak. Let the steak stand at room temperature and then turn it in the bag after thirty minutes so the steak can be well-coated.
- While the steak is marinating, cut the bell pepper into 1-inch

pieces and combine with 0.25 c of onion in water. When it is finished, just so the onions are soft. You can blend them together in a powerful blender until they are smooth. Then stir in 0.25 tsp of salt and a tablespoon of oil.

- Slice the remaining pepper and add the pepper and remaining onions to a cast iron skillet.
- Cook until the peppers are wilted. Stir in 0.25 teaspoon salt and black pepper. Remove it from the pan and keep it warm.
- Then remove the steak from the marinade and toss the marinade out.
- Then put the skillet on high heat and add the steak.
- Cook on 3 minutes on both sides until the steak is glazed on both sides. You can also cook it to your liking at this stage.
- Then cut the steak diagonally into slices and serve with the pepper and corn mixture. You can garnish with thyme if you want.

Easy Tomato Soup

This recipe takes 5 minutes to prepare, 40 minutes to cook, and it makes 6 servings.

A serving contains:

- 3 grams Protein
- 1 gram Carbohydrates
- 8 grams Total fat

What to Use

- Basil (2 tablespoons)
- Heavy cream (0.25 c, low fat if you can find it or the vegan option)
- Salt and Pepper (to taste)
- Chicken bone broth (you can choose whichever broth you want) (2 c)
- Garlic cloves (4 minced)
- Olive oil (2 tablespoons)
- Roma tomatoes (10 medium ones cut into 1" cubes)

What to Do

- Preheat the oven to about 400 degrees and lightly grease a baking sheet. Rinse the tomatoes and then chop them into cubes. Then mix the tomato chunks with minced garlic and extra-virgin olive oil.
- Roast the tomatoes for about 20-30 minutes in the oven. You can turn them about halfway through so both sides are roasted nicely.
- When they are roasted, take them out of the oven and cool
- Then put the tomatoes into a blender and puree until it is

smooth.
- Then put the tomato puree into a pot, add the broth, and season to taste. Simmer for about 15 minutes.
- Add in the fresh basil and then the cream. You can serve with toasted bread or a salad.

Salmon, Avocado, and Sweet Kale Salad with a Lemon Vinaigrette

This recipe takes 5 minutes to prepare, and it makes 6 servings.
A serving contains:

- 14 grams Fat
- 7 grams Protein
- 10 grams Total Carbs
- 7 grams Net Carbs
- 3 grams Fiber
- 4 grams Sugar

What to Use
Salmon, Avocado, and Sweet Kale Salad

- Sweet Kale Salad Mix (1 12-ounce bag)
- Smoked salmon (4-ounce cut into bite-size pieces)
- Avocado (0.5 of a medium avocado, cut in cubes)

Lemon Vinaigrette Dressing

- Mayonnaise or vegan mayo (0.25 c)
- Olive oil (1 tbsp)
- Lemon juice (1 tbsp)
- Garlic powder (0.25 tsp)
- Sweetener (2 tbsp)
- Poppy seeds (1 tsp)

What to Do

- Smoke your salmon. Then combine the salad mix and salmon in a large bowl.

- Mix all the dressing ingredients together. You can whisk it together. Then toss the dressing with the salad.
- Add cubed avocado to the salad, and then toss the salad again.
- You can also add a few pepper flakes to make it have extra heat.

Halibut and Lemon Pesto

This recipe takes 3 minutes to prepare, 8 minutes to cook, and it makes 4 servings.

A serving contains:

- 38.7 grams Protein
- 0.5 grams Fiber
- 1.4 grams Carbohydrates
- 363 milligrams Sodium
- 6.3 grams MSG
- 2.3 grams Polysaturated Fat
- 2.6 grams Saturated Fat
- 13 grams Total fat

What to Use

- Lemon juice (1 tbsp)
- Lemon rind (1 tbsp grated)
- Garlic cloves (2 peeled)
- Extra-virgin olive oil (2 tbsp)
- Fresh cheese (0.25 c)
- Basil leaves (0.66 c)
- Salt and Pepper (to taste)
- Cooking spray
- Halibut or any firm white fish (4, 6 oz filets)

What to Do

- Get your grill ready.
- Season the fish with salt and pepper. Coat the grill with cooking spray.
- Grill for at least 4 minutes on each side until flaky.

- As the fish grills, make the pesto.
- Combine a pinch of salt, basil, pepper, garlic cloves, lemon rind and lemon juice to make the pesto. And blend it all together until it is minced.
- When it is ready to serve, add a fresh squeeze of lemon juice over the top.

Dinner

Cold Cucumber Soup

This recipe takes 15 minutes to prepare and makes 4 servings
    A serving contains:

- 1 gram Protein
- 6 grams Sugar
- 2 grams Fiber
- 11 grams Carbohydrates
- 122 milligrams Potassium
- 159 milligrams Sodium
- 1 gram Fat

What to Use

- Sliced almonds (to garnish)
- Diced red pepper and cucumber (to garnish)
- Salt (0.5 teaspoon)
- Lime juice from half a lime
- Apple (1 sweet one of your choice, cored and peeled)
- Green onion (2)
- Basil Leaves (5 fresh ones)
- Garlic cloves (2)
- Unsweetened Almond Milk (1 cup)
- English cucumbers (2 or about 4 cups)

What to Do

- Blend all the ingredients together and chill. You can also serve warm.

- Add water to thin.
- When you're ready to eat it, garnish with the toppings of your choice.

Caprese Tomato Salad

This recipe takes 20 minutes to prepare, and it makes 4 servings.
A serving contains:

- 2 grams Protein
- 4 grams Sugar
- 2 grams Fiber
- 5 grams Carbohydrates
- 207 milligrams Sodium
- 2.7 grams Monosaturated fat
- 0.4 grams Polysaturated Fat
- 1.8 grams Saturated Fat
- 5.8 grams Total fat

What to Use

- Fresh mozzarella cheese (1 oz low-fat or vegan and diced)
- Salt (0.25 tsp)
- Black Pepper (0.25 tsp)
- Balsamic Vinegar (1 tbsp)
- Extra-virgin olive oil (1 tbsp)
- Basil leaves (0.5 c)
- Cherry Tomatoes (3 cups halved)
- Whole-grain bread (optional)
- Sprouted bread (optional)
- Lettuce wraps (optional)

What to Do

- Combine a pinch of salt and the tomatoes in a big bowl. Mix them all together to let the flavors fuse.
- Let it stand for 5 minutes.

- Then add in the basil leaves, balsamic vinegar, a pinch of salt and pepper, mozzarella, and toss. You can serve with fresh basil.
- If you want to make the mixture into a sandwich, you can add the mixture to a lettuce wrap or on top of your favorite whole-grain or sprouted grain bread. Or you can enjoy it on its own.

Grilled Cabbage Steaks

This recipe takes 10 minutes to prepare, 40 minutes to cook, and it makes 8 servings.

A serving contains:

- 4 grams Protein
- 3 grams Sugar
- 2 grams Fiber
- 8 grams Carbohydrates
- 15 grams Total fat

What to Use

- Black Pepper (0.5 tsp)
- Salt (0.5 tsp)
- Lemon Juice (2 tbsp)
- Olive Oil (0.25 c)
- Garlic (8 minced cloves)
- Cabbage (1 head)
- Bacon (8 slices)

What to Do

- Marinade for Cabbage Steak
- Fry the bacon and let the bacon fat cool. While the bacon is frying, cut the cabbage into 0.75-inch-thick slices. Then in a large bag, add the lemon juice, olive oil, salt, and pepper.
- When the bacon fat has cooled enough not to melt the plastic, mix all the ingredients together. Then add the sliced cabbage steaks to the marinade bag and marinate for about 30 minutes. You can switch the position after about 30 minutes so the cabbage can be marinated thoroughly.
- Preheat the grill the medium heat and grill the steaks for

about 4-8 minutes on each side until the edges are tender and crispy.

Roasted Chicken and Zucchini in One Pan

This recipe takes 15 minutes to prepare, 20 minutes to cook, and it makes 4 servings.

A serving contains:

- 37 grams Protein
- 10 grams Sugar
- 39 grams Total fat

What to Use

- Rosemary (1 tbsp)
- Zucchini (1.5 peeled and trimmed)
- Salt and Pepper (to taste)
- Extra-virgin olive Oil (4 tbsp)
- Onion (1 cut and peeled into eights)
- Chicken thighs (4)

What to Do

- Preheat the oven to 425 degrees. Put the carrots and onion in one layer on a greased baking sheet.
- Drizzle the olive oil over the vegetable and season with salt and pepper. Then add the chicken thighs that are seasoned with salt, pepper, and olive oil.
- Roast in the oven for 15-20 minutes until the skin is brown, and the carrots are tender. You can serve this with a nice salad or steamed vegetables.

Portobello Pizza

This recipe takes 10 minutes to prepare, 20 minutes to cook, and it makes 4 servings.

A serving contains:

- 6 grams Fat
- 7 grams Protein
- 5 grams Carbohydrates
- 4 grams Net Carbs
- 1 gram Fiber
- 3 grams Sugar

What to Use

- Olive oil spray
- Pepperoni or turkey or meatless sausage (16 slices)
- Portobello mushrooms (4 large ones)
- Marinara sauce (0.5 c)
- Low-fat mozzarella shredded cheese (0.5 c)

What to Do

- Preheat the oven to 375 degrees Fahrenheit. Line a baking sheet with parchment paper or aluminum foil. Coat it well with a layer of olive oil spray.
- Scrape out the dark gills from the mushrooms with a spoon, and discard the gills.
- Place the mushrooms with the stems up, and top each one with 2 tbsp of marinara sauce. Also sprinkle each with 2 tbsp low-fat mozzarella, and 4 slices of the meat you want each.
- Bake for 20 to 25 minutes, until the cheese, is bubbly, and the mushrooms are soft. You can also serve with a salad.

Snacks

Mini Zucchini Pizzas

This recipe takes minutes to prepare and minutes to cook, and it makes servings.

A serving contains:

- 2 grams Protein
- 1 gram Sugar
- 1 gram Carbohydrates
- 108 milligrams Sodium
- 1 gram Saturated Fat
- 2 grams Total fat

What to Use

- Minced basil
- Mini pepperoni or meatless mini pepperoni slices (0.5 c)
- Low-fat mozzarella or vegan cheese (0.75 c)
- Pizza sauce (0.3 c)
- Pepper (0.125 tsp)
- Salt (0.125 tsp)
- Zucchini (1 large one)

What to Do

- Cut the zucchini diagonally into 0.25-inch slices.
- Then preheat the broiler. Arrange the zucchini on a greased baking sheet or one lined with aluminum foil and sprayed with cooking spray. Keep it in one single layer.
- Broil it 3-4 inches for about 1-2 minutes on each side until the zucchini is crisp and tender.

- After you take the zucchini out, sprinkle it with salt and pepper. Then top with sauce, the pepperoni, and cheese. Broil again for about 1 minute until the cheese is melted. Sprinkle with basil if you would like.

Spinach and Turkey Pinwheels

This recipe takes minutes to prepare and minutes to cook, and it makes servings.

A serving contains:

- 17 grams Protein
- 1 gram Sugar
- 1 gram Fiber
- 31 grams Carbohydrates
- 866 milligrams Sodium
- 6 grams Saturated Fat
- 13 grams Total fat

What to Use

- Sliced Deli Turkey (1 pound)
- Fresh baby spinach (4 cups)
- Tortillas or lettuce wraps (8, 8-inch)
- Low-fat garden vegetable cream cheese (1 8oz carton)

What to Do

Spread the cream cheese over the tortillas or lettuce wraps. Then alternate and layer it with turkey and spinach. Roll it up tightly and stick a toothpick in it. You can refrigerate until it is ready to be served.

Broccoli Salad with Bacon

This recipe takes 10 minutes to prepare, and it makes 10 servings. A serving contains:

- 11 grams Fat
- 4 grams Protein
- 5 grams Total Carbohydrates
- 1.5 grams Fiber
- 1.5 grams Sugar

What to Use
Broccoli Salad

- Bacon bits (0.5 c)
- Broccoli (1 bunch, chopped into small florets)
- Red onion (0.25 c sliced)

Creamy Lemon Poppy Seed Dressing

- Garlic powder (0.5 tsp)
- Poppy seeds (0.5 tsp)
- Salt (to taste)
- Pepper (to taste)
- Mayonnaise or vegan mayo (0.5 c)
- Olive oil (1 tbsp)
- Lemon juice (1 tbsp)
- Sweetener of choice (1.5 tbsp)

What to Do

- Combine all the salad together: chopped broccoli, red onion and bacon bits, in a large bowl.
- Then in another smaller bowl, mix and whisk together the

mayonnaise, olive oil, lemon juice, garlic powder, orange zest, sweetener, and poppy seeds. Adjust the sweetener of your choice to taste. Then season it with sea salt and black pepper to taste.
- Finally, stir the dressing into the vegetable mixture. Refrigerate for an hour or more for better flavor.
- For a meatless option, go for meat-free bacon bits or forget the bacon altogether. If you do not like walnuts, you can skip them or substitute it with your favorite walnut. This would pair well with a smoothie, too.

Cauliflower Hummus

This recipe takes 10 minutes of preparation time, 40 minutes of cooking time, and it makes 4 servings.

A serving contains:

- 15 grams Fat
- 6 grams Protein
- 10 grams Total Carbohydrates
- 6 grams Fiber

What to Use

- Garlic powder (2 cloves, crushed)
- Smoked Paprika (0.5 tsp)
- Salt (1 tsp)
- Olive oil (1 tbsp)
- Tahini (0.3 c tbsp)
- Cauliflower (1 medium)
- Cumin (2 tbsp)
- Coriander (for garnish)

What to Do

- Preheat the oven to 180 degrees C. Take off all the florets from the cauliflower.
- Put the florets on a baking tray and cover them with cumin. Let them bake for 30 minutes or until a lot of the water has left the florets.
- Take it out and let the cauliflower cool. Then put it into a blender, and blend it all together until it's chunky. Then put in the paprika, salt, crushed garlic and tahini, and blend some more.
- You can serve it in a small bowl, covered with olive oil

coriander as a garnish.

Linseed or Flax Seed Crackers

This recipe takes 15 minutes to prepare, 4 hours to cook, and it makes 40 crackers.

A serving contains:

- 2 grams Fat
- 1 gram Protein
- 1 gram Total Carbohydrates
- 1 gram Fiber

What to Use
Salt (0.5 tsp)
Paprika, Smoked (0.5 tsp)
Water
Linseeds or flaxseeds (150 g)
What to Do

- Put the flax seeds in a bowl and add the salt and smoked paprika. Cover it with water until the seeds are covered. Let it sit overnight.
- Then the next day, on a large baking tray, spread out the linseed mixtures and make sure the seeds are not any deeper than 1 or 2 seeds.
- Then you can cook at about 90 degrees Celsius for 4 hours. Once the moisture has cooked out, you can take the crackers out and slice them thinly.

Conclusion

Thank for making it through to the end of *Intermittent Fasting: The Beginner's Guide for Women Who Want to Lose Weight with The Ketogenic Diet for Ultimate Weight-Loss and Fat Burning*, let's hope it was informative and able to provide you with all of the tools you need to achieve your goals whatever they may be.

Fasting is not new to humankind. From the beginning of time to modern time, the benefits of fasting have been lauded by philosophers and health practitioners alike. Some of the earliest indications of the benefits of fasting were to deal with sickness. Researchers today have shown that intermittent fasting is indeed healthy, and it has many health benefits that can help you live a long and healthy life. For Americans who are dealing with unhealthy lifestyles, intermittent fasting may just be the solution that they are looking for. The journey to intermittent fast name is an easy one to start, but maintaining it can be difficult. Whether you are afraid of not being able to make it through your fat and window or just afraid that your body will go haywire once you begin, all valid concerns, they are concerns that can be overcome if you make a slow and gradual approach to intermittent fasting. If at any point, you feel extremely concerned, reach out to your doctor. So what do you have to lose? This book has given you everything that you need to know and hopefully has alleviated any fears that you may have about intermittent fasting.

We have attempted to give you an overview of what intermittent fasting is, how it benefits your lifestyle, and why you should be doing it. The following chapters gave you an overview of what intermittent fasting and fasting is all about and how you can get started today. In Chapter one, we talked about fasting and gave a brief overview of fasting and the benefits it can have on your life. In Chapter 2, practical tips on how to fast were given, and steps were given that can help you begin. Different versions of extended fasting were explored in Chapter 3, as well as, tips to help you curb your hunger while fasting. Chapter 4 answers all the questions you may have about fasting, and Chapter 5 gives you tips that can help you begin. All the chapters demonstrate that fasting is doable, feasible, and a reasonable lifestyle choice for people who want to be healthy.

Successful Intermittent Fasting Stories

Many celebrities follow the intermittent fasting lifestyle with wonderful results. You are not the only person who knows the value of intermittent fasting. Celebrities have long been practicing intermittent fasting for years. Check out who they are and which fasting style works best for them.

- Jimmy Kimmel follows the 5:2 intermittent dieting. It has helped him maintain his weight. For him, he eats about 500 calories on Thursday and Monday. The other day, he eats what he wants. But guess what he drinks on the days that he's fasting? Yup, good ol' coffee to help him make it through the day.
- Terry Crews typically eats from 2-10 pm every day. He follows the 16:8 intermittent fasting lifestyle. He works out while fasting and feels like intermittent fasting has helped him stay in shape. He even sometimes eats a little coconut oil on a spoon to help him make it through his fast, a great tip to know. He also states that intermittent fasting has him feeling better than he was younger due to intermittent fasting's know energy boosting effects.
- Jennifer Metcalfe is another celebrity who follows the 5:2 intermittent fasting plan and notes how it helps her with her workouts and give her more energy as well.
- Hugh Jackman credits his intermittent fasting method of 16:8 as helping him maintain his weight. He also says that intermittent fasting helps him sleep well at night.

- Nicole Kidman is known to follow the 16:8 intermittent fasting method. She usually just eats lean proteins and lots of vegetables as well.
- Justin Theroux is an actor who cut out sugar and goes on about a 12 hour fast for about two to three weeks at a time. He eats from 7 am and 7 pm. He also drinks amino acids to help him curb his appetite.
- Beyoncé, although she has not confirmed due to her low-key profile, is also said to practice intermittent fasting.
- Chris Hemsworth has done the 15:9 method to lose weight for movies roles. He also eats 500-600 calories per day to lose with for roles as a weight to get as most weight loss as possible by pairing intermittent fasting and a caloric deficit.
- Benedict Cumberbatch also does the 5:20 diet and eats less than 500 calories on his fasting days to maintain his physique for his movie roles.
- Ben Affleck, Jennifer Lopez, and Miranda Kerr are also known to practice intermittent fasting.

It seems like intermittent fasting is one of the best-kept secrets that stars use to get in shape for movie roles and to maintain their weight. Thankfully, you now know the value in a minute fasting, and you can incorporate it in your life so you can be movie star ready as well.

I hope that you do not delay in starting your intermittent fasting lifestyle. The quicker you begin, the quicker you can start seeing improved health results and an improvement in overall health goals. To get even better results, you should consider doing the keto diet with your intermittent fasting. It will improve the results of intermittent fasting vastly. Learning to overcome your hunger is no joke. It is a very real concern that many people have before they begin intermittent fasting. The good news is that there are short-term strategies and long-term strategies that can help you overcome any hunger pains you may have.

The more your body gets used to your fasting windows, the easier it will be to make it through them. Overcoming hunger is mental as well as physical. If you are eating a well-balanced diet, being consistent and are determined to make it work, you will. Armed with practical, helpful ways to keep your appetite in check and curb your hunger, there is no reason why intermittent fasting isn't for you. Along with the other chapters in the book and this guide, there is no reason why you can't succeed at being intermittent faster.

So how about you? What's holding you back? No more excuses. The next step is to make a real commitment to start intermittent fasting. Decide what method you are going to use. Which window will fit best into your life as it is now? Would it be 5:3, 16:8: 12:12 or eat a day and skip a day? Whichever one it is, pick that method. Soon you will join the ends of people who know the power of intermittent fasting, and you will revel in the healthy your lifestyle that you now have thanks to the many benefits of an intermittent fasting lifestyle. When you look back at the time that you were not intermittent fasting, you will be able to laugh and smile knowing that you are now doing what you thought at one time was impossible. You will grin in the light in the fact that there is a sweetness in the stomach emptiness that you are now privy to enjoying.

Finally, if you found this book useful in any way, a review on Amazon is always appreciated!

© Copyright 2019_All rights reserved.

The following eBook is reproduced below with the goal of providing information that is as accurate and reliable as possible. Regardless, purchasing this eBook can be seen as consent to the fact that both the publisher and the author of this book are in no way experts on the topics discussed within and that any recommendations or suggestions that are made herein are for entertainment purposes only. Professionals should be consulted as needed prior to undertaking any of the action endorsed herein.

This declaration is deemed fair and valid by both the American Bar Association and the Committee of Publishers Association and is legally binding throughout the United States.

Furthermore, the transmission, duplication, or reproduction of any of the following work including specific information will be considered an illegal act irrespective of if it is done electronically or in print. This extends to creating a secondary or tertiary copy of the work or a recorded copy and is only allowed with the express written consent from the Publisher. All additional right reserved.

The information in the following pages is broadly considered a truthful and accurate account of facts and as such, any inattention, use, or misuse of the information in question by the reader will render any resulting actions solely under their purview. There are no scenarios in which the publisher or the original author of this work can be in any fashion deemed liable for any hardship or damages that may befall them after undertaking information described herein.

Additionally, the information in the following pages is intended only for informational purposes and should thus be thought of as universal. As befitting its nature, it is presented without assurance regarding its prolonged validity or interim quality. Trademarks that are mentioned are done without written consent and can in no way be considered an endorsement from the trademark holder.

---

[1] (2019)

[2] (2019)

[3] (2019)

[4] ("Success Stories", n.d.)

[5] ("9 Intermittent Fasting Weight Loss Before and After Pictures — Wise-Jug.com", n.d.)

[6] ("9 Intermittent Fasting Weight Loss Before and After Pictures — Wise-Jug.com", n.d.)

[7] ("Success Stories", n.d.)

[8] ("Success Stories", n.d.)

[9] ("Success Stories", n.d.)

[10] ("Success Stories", n.d.)

[11] ("These Experts Explain Exactly Why Intermittent Fasting Really Works", 2019)

[12] ("These Experts Explain Exactly Why Intermittent Fasting Really Works", 2019)

[13] ("These Experts Explain Exactly Why Intermittent Fasting Really Works", 2019)

[14] ("27 Keto Diet Before-And-After Photos That Will Make Your Jaw Drop", n.d.)

[15] ("27 Keto Diet Before-And-After Photos That Will Make Your Jaw Drop", n.d.)

[16] ("27 Keto Diet Before-And-After Photos That Will Make Your Jaw Drop", n.d.)

[17] ("27 Keto Diet Before-And-After Photos That Will Make Your Jaw Drop", n.d.)

[18] ("27 Keto Diet Before-And-After Photos That Will Make Your Jaw Drop", n.d.)

[19] ("27 Keto Diet Before-And-After Photos That Will Make Your Jaw Drop", n.d.)

[20] ("27 Keto Diet Before-And-After Photos That Will Make Your Jaw Drop", n.d.)

[21] ("27 Keto Diet Before-And-After Photos That Will Make Your Jaw Drop", n.d.)

[22] (Åkesson & Dr. Andreas Eenfeldt, 2018)

[23] ("Keto Success Stories", n.d.)

[24] ("Keto Success Stories", n.d.)

[25] (Åkesson & Dr. Andreas Eenfeldt, 2019)

[26] (Åkesson & Dr. Andreas Eenfeldt, 2019)

[27] (Åkesson & Dr. Andreas Eenfeldt, 2019)

[28] (Åkesson & Dr. Andreas Eenfeldt, 2019)

[29] (Åkesson & Dr. Andreas Eenfeldt, 2019)

[30] ("Ketosis Explained: What It Is, How to Achieve It (And Why You Want To)", n.d.)

www.ingramcontent.com/pod-product-compliance
Lightning Source LLC
LaVergne TN
LVHW020429070526
838199LV00004B/327